Exercise Dependence

D0282294

Exercise dependence has been described as a 'positive addiction', but it can have links with damaging dysfunctional and excessive behaviours, including eating disorders. Clinical and sport psychologists now acknowledge the condition and report that it can be found in both recreational exercisers and competitive athletes.

This is the first text to provide a comprehensive review of exercise dependence. The text contains case studies and reviews research in both 'exercise' and 'sports' contexts. The authors examine the condition in the widest sense, exploring different types of exercise dependence, risk factors associated with the condition, the experiences and motivational characteristics of sufferers, links with eating disorders, and a number of approaches to counselling.

This text will be of significant interest to psychologists working in sport, health and clinical practice, as well as to athletes and sports coaches, particularly those involved in endurance sports associated with higher incidences of exercise dependence.

John H. Kerr is Professor of Sport Psychology in the Faculty of Sport and Physical Education, Kokushikan University, Japan.

Koenraad J. Lindner is Senior Lecturer in Sport Psychology, retired, from the University of Hong Kong, China.

Michelle Blaydon has a PhD in Sports Psychology and is a senior research analyst for a commercial organization.

Exercise Dependence

John H. Kerr, Koenraad J. Lindner
and Michelle Blaydon

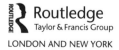

LONDON AND NEW YORK

First published 2007
by Routledge
2 Park Square, Milton Park, Abingdon, Oxon OX14 4RN

Simultaneously published in the USA and Canada
by Routledge
270 Madison Ave, New York, NY 10016

*Routledge is an imprint of the Taylor & Francis Group,
an informa business*

Typeset in Goudy by
Florence Production Ltd, Stoodleigh, Devon
Printed and bound in Great Britain by
TJ International Ltd, Padstow, Cornwall

Every effort has been made to ensure that the advice and
information in this book is true and accurate at the time of going
to press. However, neither the publisher nor the author can accept
any legal responsibility or liability for any errors or omissions that
may be made. In the case of drug administration, any medical
procedure or the use of technical equipment mentioned within
this book, you are strongly advised to consult the manufacturer's
guidelines.

British Library Cataloguing in Publication Data
A catalogue record for this book is available
from the British Library

Library of Congress Cataloging in Publication Data
Kerr, J. H.
   Exercising dependence/John H. Kerr, Koenraad J. Lindner
   and Michelle Blaydon.
       p. cm.
       Includes bibliographical references and indexes.
   1. Exercise addiction.   I. Lindner, Koenraad J., 1941–
   II. Blaydon, Michelle.   III. Title.
   [DNLM: 1. Behavior, Addictive – psychology. 2. Exercise –
   psychology. WM 176 K41e 2007]
   RC569.5E94K47 2007
   616.85'2 – dc22   2007003800

ISBN13: 978–0–415–39344–7 (hbk)
ISBN13: 978–0–415–39345–4 (pbk)
ISBN13: 978–0–203–94679–4 (ebk)

ISBN10: 0–415–39344–2 (hbk)
ISBN10: 0–415–39345–0 (pbk)
ISBN10: 0–203–94679–0 (ebk)

The antithesis of exercise dependence: 'Whenever I feel like exercise I lie down until the feeling passes.' (Robert M. Hutchins – American educator)

Contents

Figures and tables

Figures

Tables

Preface

Anyone who needs to understand the power that a dependency or addiction can hold over a person need look no further than some examples from among the world's elite sportsmen. Take, for example, former National Basketball Association star player and current TV analyst Charles Barkley. He averaged 22.1 points per game in a sixteen-year career with teams in Philadelphia, Phoenix, and Houston, and he was the NBA's most valuable player in 1993. He also won a gold medal with the US 'Dream Team' in the Barcelona Olympics. In 2006, Barkley admitted that, although he had never bet on NBA games, he had probably lost about $10 million through gambling in casinos, betting as much as $20,000 a hand.

John Daly, professional golfer, has had problems with both gambling and alcohol. Daly won two major tournaments, including the 1995 British Open at St Andrews, and five Professional Golfers' Association (PGA) tour victories, as well as the PGA championship in 1991. He said, in the final chapter of his autobiography, *John Daly: my life in and out of the rough*, that he had lost between $50 and $60 million during twelve years of heavy gambling. On one occasion, after earning $750,000 when he lost in a playoff to Tiger Woods at a 2005 World Golf Championship game in San Francisco, he drove to Las Vegas instead of going home, and lost $1.65 million in five hours, mostly playing $5,000 slot machines. After playing one round at the Players Championship in March 1997, he was forced to withdraw after a drunken spree in which he caused more than $1,000 worth of damage to his hotel room. As a result, he lost a $10 million endorsement contract with a major equipment company that no longer wished to be associated with him. At around the same time, his wife filed for divorce. In 1997, Daly entered an alcohol treatment centre for the second time in four years.

Recent England international players Paul Gascoigne and Tony Adams are just two more from a long list of examples from top-flight football (soccer). Perhaps the most tragic case, however, was that of the late George Best. Best, a legendary Manchester United and Northern Ireland player and an outstanding football player of the late 1960s, has often been compared to the world's best players, Pele, Cruyff and Maradona. The highlight of his career was the two excellent goals he scored in the 1968 European Cup final in Manchester United's 5–1 win over Benfica. At the age of 22 he was at his greatest when he won the English and European Footballer of the Year awards. However, four years later, aged 26, Best retired prematurely from the game. He made several comebacks, none of which was really successful because, despite his talent, he loved the champagne and playboy lifestyle and he became an alcoholic. His personal life became problematic; bankruptcy, convictions for drunk driving and assaulting a policeman and a man in a London pub – along with broken marriages – all followed over the years before his death. Best received a liver transplant in 2002, but continued his drinking and died of multiple organ failure in 2005 at the age of 59. Best's story provides a very powerful example of how a dependency or addiction can affect an elite sports performer.

Exercise, although often thought of in more positive terms, can have just as serious an impact as alcohol and gambling on the lives of those who become addicted to it. As with the other substances and activities often associated with addictions, exercise can totally take over people's lives, affecting their working, social and family lives. This book is about *exercise dependence*.

While elite sports performers may become addicted to a substance or activity that interferes with their participation, exercise dependence actually drives people, and not just elite sports people, to exercise more and more often and for longer and longer periods. This is illustrated by the anecdote of a hospital patient who persisted in going for a run even though wired up to a drip (Startup, 2001). One of the intriguing questions about people who may become addicted to exercise to the point where they are prepared to endure extreme physical discomfort, making increasingly extreme demands on their bodies at possible risk to their health, is: 'Why do they do it? What can possibly be their motivation?'

The aim of this book is to try to provide the answer to this question, explaining how this extreme form of behaviour occurs and why it is similar to other forms of dependency and addiction, such as those mentioned above. It includes a broadly based and comprehensive update of what is currently known about exercise dependence across a number of sport and exercise contexts. In addition, it discusses important terms and definitions and uses interesting interview material and case studies to illustrate the arguments being presented. It also summarizes the current debate in the literature about the existence of exercise dependence and its links with eating disorders. To the authors' knowledge this is the first book to deal exclusively with exercise dependence, and it is our hope that it will make an important contribution to a relatively new area of study.

Information provided in this preface is taken from these sources:

Barkley, Charles (2006) 'I've blown $10 million gambling', *The Japan Times*, 5 May, p. 11.

Daly, John (2006) 'Gambling may "flat-out ruin" me', *The Japan Times*, 3 May, p. 18.

Japan Times (2005) 'Tributes pour in for Best', 27 November, p. 20.

New York Times (1997) 'Daly to enter alcohol treatment center', 31 March (archive).

New York Times (1997) 'Daly's wife seeks divorce', 11 April (archive).

Startup, H. (2001) 'Eating disorders in sport', *The Psychologist*, p. 312–13.

Acknowledgements

We would like to express our thanks to Mike Apter, George Wilson and Mieke Mitchell for their insightful comments on early drafts of the various book chapters, and to Mieke for her invaluable copyediting. Thanks are also due to Samantha Grant, Ygraine Cadlock and the rest of the publication team at Routledge for their cooperation.

The authors are also grateful to: BMJ Publishing Group Ltd, British Psychological Society Publications, John Wiley & Sons Limited, Open University Press/McGraw-Hill Publishing Co. and Routledge/Taylor & Francis Group LLC, for permission to reproduce material (specific details are included in the text).

Abbreviations

ACSM	American College of Sports Medicine
AN	anorexia nervosa
ANOVA	Analysis of Variance
APA	American Psychiatric Association
BED	binge eating disorder
BMI	body mass index
BN	bulimia nervosa
BSI	Brief Symptom Inventory
BSQ	Body Shape Questionnaire
CRQ	Commitment to Running Questionnaire
DSM	Diagnostic and Statistical Manual
EAI	Exercise Addiction Inventory
EAT	Eating Attitudes Test
EBQ	Exercise Belief Questionnaire
EDEQ	Eating Disorder Examination Questionnaire
EDI	Eating Disorder Inventory
EDNOS	eating disorder not otherwise specified
EDQ	Exercise Dependence Questionnaire
EDS	Exercise Dependence Scale
EPQ	Eysenck Personality Questionnaire
ER	endurance running
EXDI	Exercise Dependence Interview
GHQ	General Health Questionnaire
LTEQ	Leisure-Time Exercise Questionnaire
MANOVA	Multivariate Analysis of Variance
MSP	Motivational Style Profile
MSP-SE	Motivational Style Profile for Sport and Exercise
NBA	National Basketball Association
NCAA	National College Athletic Association
NCCMH	National Collaboration Centre for Mental Health
NEO-FFI	NEO Five Factor Inventory
NEO-PI-R	NEO Personality Inventory – Revised
PGA	Professional Golfers' Association

POMS	Profile of Mood States
PWB	psychological well-being
RAS	Running Addiction Scale
RSES	Rosenberg Self-Esteem Scale
SACL	Stress-Arousal Checklist
SEI	Culture Free Self-Esteem Inventory
SOMIFA	State of Mind Indicator for Athletes
SSS	Sensation Seeking Scale
TESI	Tension and Effort Stress Inventory
TSM	Telic State Measure

1 Over the top

An introduction to exercise dependence

'Addicted? Yeah. I'm addicted to it. I just can't give it up'.

'Two years ago I was weaned off it, but I know it's always there, always lurking.'

'At its best, it just gives you a sensation of being so alive and so on form. It's just, it's as though you could not be enjoying your life more at that minute.'

'I often cancelled trips and cancelled visits to friends because it meant I couldn't get this high.'

These quotes come not from alcoholics, compulsive gamblers, heroin, crack or other drug addicts but from a number of people who featured in a BBC television programme called *Fit to Drop* that was part of the *Forty Minutes* series (BBC 1990). These people were all self-confessed exercise addicts, and some were those who had given up, struggled with great difficulty to give up or at least to cut down on their exercise activities. Exercise addiction or dependence is now well recognized among sport and exercise and some clinical psychologists. Although Glasser (1976) talked about exercise as a 'positive addiction' some thirty years ago and there have been some studies and writing on the topic in the succeeding years (e.g. De Coverly Veale, 1987; Morgan, 1979; Sachs and Pargman, 1979), it was only in the early 1990s that clinical and sport psychologists began to report increasing numbers of individuals who appeared to be addicted to, or dependent on, exercise (e.g. Annett *et al.*, 1995; Pierce, 1994). Some of these individuals appeared to exhibit dysfunctional eating as well as excessive exercising behaviour (e.g. Long *et al.*, 1993; Yates, 1991).

A recent research publication from biological anthropology provides a possible explanation of why human beings are predisposed to engage in long distance running and other endurance activities. In an intriguing paper published in the prestigious journal *Nature*, biologist Dennis Bramble and biological anthropologist Daniel Lieberman examined the role of running in human evolution (Bramble and Lieberman, 2004). Rather than focusing on walking, which has been relatively well researched, these two scientists took a novel approach by examining the physiological and anatomical bases of endurance running in humans. Although humans are relatively mediocre performers when it comes to sprinting, the authors presented a range of evidence that, they argued, suggested that sustained long distance endurance using aerobic metabolism 'is a derived capability of the genus *Homo*, originating about two million years ago, and may have been instrumental in the evolution of the human body form' (Bramble and Lieberman, 2004, p. 345).

According to Bramble and Lieberman (2004), the evidence suggests that when compared with other primates humans are unique in their ability to perform endurance running. No other primate can run the sustainable distances that are covered by thousands of physically fit regular amateur runners and joggers every year. In addition, humans are able to make continuous adjustments to a wide range of running speeds without changing gait or incurring metabolic penalty.

After reviewing the considerable physiological, anatomical and fossil evidence that exists concerning the energetics, strength, stabilization and thermoregulation demands of human endurance running (ER), the authors stated that:

> Considering all the evidence together, it is reasonable to hypothesize that *Homo* evolved to travel long distances by both walking and running. New fossils and more detailed analysis of the existing fossil record are needed to test whether these two locomotor capabilities emerged concurrently or whether ER evolved after selection for long-distance walking. An even more difficult task is to determine what behaviours selected for ER in the first place. Why would early *Homo* run long distances when walking is easier, safer and less costly? One possibility is that ER played a role in helping hominids exploit protein-rich resources such as meat, marrow and brain first evident in the archaeological record at approximately 2.6 Myr ago, coincident with the first appearance of *Homo*.
>
> (Bramble and Lieberman, 2004, p. 351)

The evidence presented by Bramble and Lieberman (2004) is impressive: if they are correct in their conclusions, it is hardly surprising that nowadays a whole variety of running and other endurance exercise events, such as triathlons, take place all over the world each year. Some of these are individual efforts that try to 'break new ground' or set long distance records; others have become regular, often annual, organized events.

Take, for example, 53-year-old German extreme runner Achim Heukemes, who by himself completed a 4,568-kilometre run from the west to the east coast of Australia in 2005 in slightly more than 43 days, averaging over 100 kilometres per day (*Japan Times*, 2005), or 35-year-old Briton Bob Brown who, with five other runners, competed in the Run Across America 2004 'race' from the west to the east coast of the US. Brown finished the 4,960 kilometres in just over 21 days and was over 60 hours ahead of the next finisher (*Guardian Unlimited*, 2004; Run Across America, 2004).

There are also plenty of examples of organized annual endurance events to choose from. One is the Western States 100-Mile Endurance Run (e.g. Weinberg, 1998), which takes place in conjunction with the 100-Mile Trevis Cup Horse Race from Squaw Valley to Auburn in California. In 1974, one of the horse riders who had decided to try and complete the race on foot did so successfully in 23 hours and 42 minutes. Three years later, in 1977, with fourteen starters and three finishers, the endurance run was established in its own right. Weinberg (1998) used the runners participating in the race to gather data on her study of motivation in ultra-distance runners (races over the standard marathon distance [26 miles 385 yards or 42.2 kilometres] are considered to be ultra-distance events). As part of that study, she provided a good description of her observations at the end of the 1997 race:

> At 4:30 a.m., I went down to the stadium and watched several people just make the 24-hour cut-off for their silver belt buckle. One barely made it – another missed by only seconds!
>
> The runners I saw finish looked strong and happy, but very, very tired. Most had a cold, tired, hungry family member waiting for them. Many had friends and kids who ran the finish lap around the stadium with them. Nearly all had smiles when they finished as they were greeted by the race directors and medals were placed around their necks. Just as I had witnessed at Devil's Thumb, however, as the day wore on, people looked more and more distressed as they finished. Many staggered across the finish line and were immediately helped to cots where they received medical attention. The extraordinary courage, determination, aches and pains, willfulness, and joy of accomplishment in finishing the race were truly inspiring.
>
> (Weinberg, 1998, p. 7–8)

It is a long way from hot sunny California to the more-often-than-not cold, wet mountain peaks of the Lake District in the north of England and the Borrowdale Fell Race. The race is much shorter than the Western States 100-Mile Endurance Run; it is usually about 17 miles, and each year approximately 200 of Britain's estimated 5,000 fell runners take part (*Independent*, 2004). Fell racing dates back to the early twentieth century. Fell runners have to contend in all weathers with slow, steep climbs that continue for miles at a time and fast, steep descents. Underfoot, the ground conditions are treacherous, with loose stones, wet grass, mud and slippery rocks, made worse by the short undergrowth of heather or bracken, and the terrain is frequently engulfed in cloud. Falls and major injuries are a constant threat. Yet, in spite of the conditions, it remains an extremely popular, albeit minor sport among devotees in England (*Independent*, 2004).

Those individuals who are drawn to endurance events are, of course, not restricted to running. Sports such as cycling and swimming, for example, also lend themselves to endurance events, and they have even been combined with running to form what has become known as triathlon. Triathlon races usually comprise a combination of swimming, cycling and running, in that order, and a competitor's time includes the 'transition time' for changing shoes, collecting bikes and other necessary tasks between the three stages of the race.

The Hawaii Ironman was the first major triathlon event and now ranks as the most prestigious triathlon event in the world. It began in 1978 when three existing Hawaii endurance races were combined. These were the Waikiki Roughwater Swim (3.8 kilometres, 2.4 miles), the Around-Oahu Bike Race (180 kilometres, 112 miles, originally a two-day event) and the Honolulu Marathon (42 kilometres, 26.2 miles). In the new Ironman race, these events had to be completed in succession. A total of 12 out of 15 men finished the first race and the winner's time was 11 hours, 46 minutes and 58 seconds. The following year, the first Ironwoman finished in fifth place. In just a few years, print and television media coverage made the race so well known that organizers had to restrict entries by means of nationally organized Ironman qualifying events in other countries, and the Ironman race began to attract commercial sponsorship.

Twenty-five years later, winning times are close to 8 hours 20 minutes for men and 9 hours for women. Age groups have become a feature of the race, with competitors in their seventies included, and in 2002 an 84-year-old entrant became the Ironman's oldest competitor. Each year the race has almost 1,500 finishers and they compete for over $400,000 in prize money (Ironman, 2005). In parallel with developments in the Ironman race, interest in triathlons in general has exploded in recent years. There are now a number of different variations in existence, and these include Olympic Distance, Half Ironman, Long Distance and Sprint Distance triathlons, in which the distances to be covered by athletes vary. Other variations of triathlons consist of cross-country skiing, mountain biking and running, or swimming, mountain biking and trail running.

Whether as part of organized competitive events or individual pursuits, the types of sports described above have been chosen deliberately because it is in these activities (running, swimming, cycling, triathlons) that individuals who are addicted to or dependent on exercise are likely to be found (e.g. Annett et al., 1995; Blaydon et al., 2002; Chapman and DeCastro, 1990; Kerr, 1997; Pierce et al., 1993; Veale, 1995). This is not to say that exercise dependence or addiction cannot be found in association with other sport or exercise activities, for example, weight training and body building (Seheult, 1995), aerobics (Cohen, 1995), or mountain biking, (Cripps, 1995).

At this point, however, we must examine just what is meant by the terms 'exercise dependence' or 'exercise addiction'. In order to arrive at a clear statement of what exercise dependence or addiction actually is, it is necessary to take a more general look at how psychologists and others have used the terms when referring to other forms of dependencies or addictions (e.g. gambling, sex, alcohol, tobacco and other drugs).

Addiction and dependence

A huge literature on addiction and dependence in general exists, and it soon becomes apparent that there is widespread disagreement about whether the term 'addiction' or 'dependence' should be used and which particular activities then qualify as either addictions or dependencies. Publications by Brown (1997) and Orford (2001) are especially useful in pinning down the issues involved and trying to come up with some satisfactory solutions. Both are agreed that the field of addictions has expanded in recent years, beyond notions of chemical dependency or substance abuse, to include activities such as gambling, which have no obvious physiological basis. Indeed, some authors (e.g. Witman *et al.*, 1987) have listed as many as 40 activities that are potentially addictive. However, Brown (1997) was being both cautionary and critical when he stated:

> None of these 'new' addictions fit the simple 'chemical dependency' and substance abuse model . . . such a narrow conception of addiction is useless in understanding a whole range of psychological and social problems such as gambling or sexual excesses.
>
> (Brown, 1997, pp. 14–15)

Brown (1997) wanted not only to clarify the boundaries between what was truly addictive behaviour and what was not but also to reject the medical model concept of dependency, preferring a wider or more flexible concept of 'addictions', and he incorporated this concept into his theoretical model of behavioural addictions (Brown, 1997).

Orford (2001) was also concerned about the focus of those working in the addiction field on 'substances' and the fact that the terms 'addiction' and 'dependency' have become overly identified with drugs. In an effort to move beyond the traditional thinking associated with the term 'dependency', he suggested that the term 'addiction' was still appropriate but that the term 'excessive appetite' might actually be more accurate. He stated that:

> Although the commonplace term 'addiction' remains as apt as before, for scientists preferring a more exact term, 'excessive appetite' defines the field rather than 'drug dependence'. It is not to 'substances' that we are at risk of becoming addicted, but rather to 'objects and activities' of which drugs are a special example. This new perspective allows different comparisons to be made, new concepts to be privileged and arguably a more comprehensive and satisfactory model to be developed of how people's appetites can become out of control.
>
> (Orford, 2001, p. 2)

Orford (2001) went on to point out that labels and definitions should take into consideration the history, culture, social position and moral values associated with a person's addictive activity. 'Medical' or 'disease' labels such as 'alcoholism' or 'compulsive gambling' are unable to do this. For this reason, Orford (2001) distanced himself from the term 'dependency' and preferred to use 'excessive appetite', 'strong attachment' and 'addiction', terms that, by his own admission, he used interchangeably (Orford, 2001, p. 347). He thought these latter three terms were advantageous because:

> They refer to circumstances in which people's activities have got them into serious conflict and trouble, but only because an appetite has grown to the point where it exceeds what is acceptable, or an attachment has become stronger to the point of significantly eroding freedom of choice.
> (Orford, 2001, p. 347)

However, as Orford (2001, p. 347) also conceded: 'No precise definition of addiction or dependence, however arbitrary, will serve all people in all places, at all times.'

A more detailed examination of Brown's (1997) and Orford's (2001) behavioural models of addiction will be undertaken in Chapter 2.

Exercise dependence or exercise addiction?

The difficulties and problems with definitions of terms that beset the addictions field in general are also present in the sport and exercise literature. Virtually all of the wide range of terms available from general psychology have been used, for example: 'compulsive', 'excessive', or 'obligatory' exercise; 'over-exercising'; 'exercise dependence'; 'exercise addiction'; 'positive' or 'negative exercise addiction'; 'committed runners' and 'running addiction' (Szabo, 2000). In this book, the terms *exercise dependence* and *exercise addiction* will be used interchangeably, with the understanding that both terms represent the broader interpretation of the terms advocated by Brown (1997) and Orford (2001).

Some authors have expressed their reservations about whether exercise dependence really exists or whether it is a myth (e.g. Keski-Rahkonen, 2001). Others are convinced that it does exist. Whiting (1994) provided a useful definition:

> Exercise addiction is characterized by dependency on physical activity in one or more of its forms, and by withdrawal symptoms if participation is denied. Dependency manifests itself in an excessive dominance of exercise in everyday life, often to the detriment of other facets such as the family, social contacts or work. Withdrawal symptoms include, on the psychological front, feelings of nervousness, guilt, anxiety and lowered self-esteem and, on the physiological front, headaches and physical discomfort.
> (Whiting 1994, cited in Cripps, 1995, p. 22)

In the US, Hausenblas and Giacobbi (2004) defined exercise dependence as 'a craving for physical activity that results in extreme exercise and generates negative physiological (e.g. overuse injuries, tolerance) and psychological symptoms (e.g. negative affect when unable to exercise; Hausenblas & Symons Downs, 2002a)' (Hausenblas and Giacobbi, 2004, p. 1265).

These two definitions are rather similar, but a further distinction has been made between exercise dependence occurring on its own and exercise dependence occurring in conjunction with an eating disorder. Veale (1995) considered this distinction important and called the former 'primary exercise dependence' and the latter 'secondary exercise dependence'. From his clinical experience, he considered secondary exercise dependence to be far more common than the primary version (Veale, 1995, p. 1). He proposed some operational criteria for what he called primary exercise dependence:

(1) Preoccupation with exercise which has become stereotyped and routine.
(2) Significant withdrawal symptoms in the absence of exercise (for example mood swings, irritability, insomnia).
(3) The preoccupation causes clinically significant distress or impairment in their physical, social, occupational or other important areas of functioning.
(4) The preoccupation with exercise is not better accounted for by another mental disorder (e.g. as a means of losing weight or controlling calorie intake as in an eating disorder).

(Veale, 1995, p. 2)

Veale's (1995) criteria share a good deal of common ground with the criteria developed by Brown (1993) for a range of drug and non-drug addictions. Hausenblas and Symons Downs (2002b) argued that Veale's criteria, which loosely followed the style of the criteria used in the Diagnostic and Statistical Manual (DSM-IV; American Psychiatric Association, 1994) criteria for 'substance abuse' and 'disorders of impulse control', should be expanded to follow DSM-IV criteria more closely. They recommended that:

exercise dependence be operationalized as a multidimensional maladaptive pattern of exercise, leading to clinically significant impairment or distress, as manifested by *three or more* of the following: (1) *tolerance*: which is defined as either a need for significantly increased amounts of exercise to achieve the desired effect or diminished effect with continued use of the same amount of exercise; (2) *withdrawal*: as manifested by either withdrawal symptoms for exercise (e.g. anxiety, fatigue) or the same (or closely related) amount of exercise is taken to relieve or avoid withdrawal symptoms; (3) *intention effects*: exercise is often taken in larger amounts or over a longer period than was intended; (4) *loss of control*: there is a persistent desire or unsuccessful effort to cut down or control exercise: (5) *time*: a great deal of time is spent in activities necessary to obtain exercise (e.g. vacations are exercise related); (6) *conflict*: important social, occupational, or recreational activities are given up or reduced because of exercise; and (7) *continuance*: exercise is continued despite knowledge of having a persistent or recurrent physical or psychological problem that is likely to have been caused or exacerbated by the exercise (e.g. continued running despite severe shin splints).

(Hausenblas and Symons Downs, 2002b, p. 113)[1]

There is continued discussion about the validity of the distinction between primary and secondary exercise dependence (e.g. Bamber *et al.*, 2000; Cox and Orford, 2004). While the association between exercise dependence and eating disorders (secondary dependence) has been known for some time (e.g. Yates, 1991), the results of recent research findings indicate that primary exercise dependence does exist as a separate entity (e.g. Blaydon *et al.*, 2004; Griffiths, 1997; Veale, 1995). Veale (1995; primary) and Yates (1991; secondary) have provided good examples of the two types of exercise dependence:

She was a 27-year-old single unemployed woman who was a graduate in recreation management. She had responded to an advertisement in a local sports club requesting volunteers for a study of people who considered themselves addicted to exercise. She had not previously sought help for any emotional or behavioural problem related to her exercise. She was training to be a marathon runner and had a personal best of 2 hours 40 minutes. Her weekly routine consisted of cycling 15 miles a day and twice-daily runs except on Sundays (average 14 miles) and Wednesdays (10 miles). She also did weight training twice a week.

When I saw her, the total amount of her running was not excessive but she had no other interests in life. She described her running as a compulsion ('I've got to do it'). She would experience withdrawal symptoms consisting of depressed mood, insomnia, restlessness, and indecisiveness when she had been forced to reduce her training because of an injury. She had once taken two overdoses in five days when she was withdrawing. She had presented to the Casualty Department but had not received any psychiatric help. She described her aims in life as 'to run till I die' and to represent her country in the Olympics. One of the most striking aspects of her history was that she continued to exercise through back pain. On one occasion, she had run a marathon with a fever from German measles; on another occasion when she had a fever she had stopped after 16 miles. She had lost her partner because of her exercise and there were frequent arguments with her family about the amount of time she was spending exercising and the damage to her health. She did not work because it interfered with her training.

(Veale, 1995, p. 3)[2]

Patty is a 31-year-old married woman who describes herself as 'a serious runner who does not know enough to quit'. She runs more than 200 miles a month and also bicycles 200–250 miles a week. She has sustained two serious stress fractures. Before her tibula [sic] broke, she had been in pain for months but continued to run. She carefully measures time and distance and resets her goals so that they are greater than her current performance.

Patty became a serious runner in part because the faster she became, the more weight she lost. She is 5'7" and once weighed 150 lbs, at which time she felt 'gross'. Now she weighs 115 and would like to get down to 110. She runs at least eight miles every day in order to balance out the food she ate the day before. If she overeats, she runs extra miles to get it off. She may use laxatives or give herself an enema before a race. Until six months ago, she was inducing emesis at least once a week because she was afraid of gaining weight, but now she uses only exercise and feels in total control of her body.

(Yates, 1991, p. 39)[3]

Is there a physiological basis to exercise dependence?

Earlier in this chapter, it was suggested that important anthropological and biological research findings indicated that endurance running played an important role in human evolution from the days of early *Homo* (Bramble and Lieberman, 2004). These findings, which examined the physiological and anatomical bases of endurance running in humans, might help to explain both current human involvement in endurance events and why humans enjoy these events so much, to the extent that some become dependent on exercise. In short, there may be an underlying anthropological and biological connection to explain exercise dependence. If this connection does exist, does it also include the release of chemicals in the pleasure centres of the brain?

It is often reported anecdotally that people who are addicted to running or other forms of exercise have become hooked on an 'adrenaline high'. These statements seem to be based on a kind of 'gut instinct' rather than scientific fact. However, research studies have been carried out that have examined a possible physiological basis to exercise dependence. Murphy (1994), for example, reviewed the evidence for three physiological hypotheses that have been put forward to explain the pleasant feelings that often accompany participation for regular exercisers. She examined: (1) the *thermogenic effect* (increases in body temperature with exercise reduce tonic muscle activity and then somatic anxiety); (2) the *catecholamine hypothesis* (exercise activates the release of catecholamines [including adrenaline, noradrenaline and dopamine], which are then thought to bring about feelings of euphoria and positive mood states); (3) the *endorphin hypothesis* (endorphins have similar effects to opiate drugs and, when elevated by exercise, lead to increases in pleasant mood states). In each case, Murphy admitted that the research findings were inconclusive, and the three hypotheses remain unproven and speculative, though they may still be plausible. This is a position shared by others (e.g. Loumidis and Roxborough, 1995; Steinberg *et al.*, 1995). Szabo (2000) described a fourth hypothesis, first proposed by Thompson and Blanton (1987), the *sympathetic arousal hypothesis*:

> According to this model, regular exercise leads to decreased sympathetic arousal at rest. This adaptation leads to a lethargic state with lack of exercise. To maintain an optimal level of arousal, and to overcome the lethargic state at rest, the habituated exerciser needs to exercise to increase her/his level of arousal.
>
> (Szabo, 2000, p. 137)

He argued that the associated symptoms match the symptoms of exercise dependence and therefore the explanation may also be plausible. The results of future research may clarify the validity of these hypotheses.

Measuring exercise dependence

In addition to matching individual symptoms and behaviour with a set of criteria in clinical work as described above, several questionnaire measures that purport to measure exercise dependence have been developed. Although this was a useful development, a number of general problems with these questionnaires have been identified (e.g. Hausenblas and Symons Downs, 2002a), for example, criticisms that measures 'indirectly' measured addiction through withdrawal symptoms; had too specific a focus, that is, were limited to one activity (e.g. running); failed to provide an operational definition of exercise addiction, thus bringing their validity into question; failed to distinguish between primary and secondary dependence; were data-driven and may thus have inherited problems by borrowing items from previous scales; were not theory-driven and thus had no conceptual basis. Some examples of these exercise dependence measures are described below.

The earliest measures concentrated on symptoms and mood states associated with withdrawal from exercise (Baekeland, 1970; Robbins and Joseph, 1985; Thaxton, 1982). Participants were either asked to project what their feelings would be if they were prevented from exercising or required to actually withdraw from exercise and have their symptoms and mood states monitored during the period of withdrawal. However, although these studies did find mood disturbances associated with exercise deprivation, they were subject to criticism on several levels, the main criticism being that they measured exercise dependence indirectly (e.g. Szabo, 1998).

One of the first attempts to construct a 'direct' exercise dependence measure was the 11-item Running Addiction Scale (RAS) developed by Chapman and De Castro (1990). It has been used in research (e.g. Aidman and

Woollard, 2003), but this scale is limited by the fact that it was directed only at running. In addition, the term 'addiction' was not operationally defined, and evaluation was based on relatively small numbers, thus making the validity of the measure questionable (Hausenblas and Symons Downs, 2002a).

Ogden *et al.* (1997) pioneered the 29-item Exercise Dependence Questionnaire (EDQ), which targeted the distinction between primary and secondary exercise dependence by including questions designed to screen for eating disordered behaviour as well as exercise dependence items. The measure also contains some items concerned with exercise withdrawal symptoms. However, Ogden *et al.* (1997) did not suggest a diagnostic cut-off score for determining exercise dependence as a possible pathological disorder (this was confirmed by D. Veale, personal communication, 12 October 2005), and this is a limitation recognized by some researchers who have used the scale (e.g. Bamber *et al.*, 2000; Blaydon *et al.*, 2002). Some questions have also been raised about the validity and internal consistency of a few items (Hausenblas and Symons Downs, 2002a).

Due to the limitations they identified in other measures, Hausenblas and Symons Downs (2002b) developed the 21-item Exercise Dependence Scale (EDS) directly from DSM-IV criteria for substance abuse. Using this scale, respondents can be categorized into 'at risk for exercise dependence', 'non-dependent-symptomatic', or 'non-dependent-asymptomatic' groups. One limitation of this scale is that it does not distinguish between primary and secondary exercise dependence. It may also be criticized for its basis on what Brown (1997) and Orford (2001) might consider a somewhat limited concept of addiction (i.e. substance abuse and the medical model). Research using this scale has just begun (e.g. Hausenblas and Giacobbi, 2004).

A recently developed measure, the short form of the Exercise Addiction Inventory (EAI: Terry *et al.*, 2004), which has just six items and is designed as a brief screening tool for identifying people at risk from primary exercise dependence, differs from the instruments described above in that it is theory-driven. It is based on Brown's (1993) general components of addiction and Griffith's application of these to the study of behaviours involved in, for example, exercise, sex, gambling, video games and the internet (Griffiths, 1996, 1997, 2002). It also specifies a cut-off point for individuals at risk of exercise addiction that represents scores in the top 15 per cent of the total score.

In spite of a number of disadvantages associated with the exercise dependence measures, there has been an encouraging progression of new scales over the last few years. This has led to the development of more sophisticated and sensitive measures. However, this process is still ongoing and some further refinement of measures will be necessary before exercise dependence can be measured with complete confidence. Further discussion of the problem of deciding on cut-off points in the EDQ, and their validity of them, will take place in later chapters. Research work using the EDQ will be examined in detail in Chapter 6.

Closing comments

One of the intriguing questions about people who may become addicted to exercise is: 'What rewards can be so special that these people are prepared to push their bodies to the limit and endure extreme physical discomfort and sometimes exercise when injured?' By the end of this book, many of the important issues about exercise addiction will have been discussed and the answer to this question should be clear. As a first step, this opening chapter has introduced the topic of exercise dependence and prepared the ground for a more detailed examination in later chapters. This examination begins in the next chapter, which outlines some of the most pertinent theoretical explanations of how people become dependent on exercise. These theories are general theories of behavioural addictions that have been applied, with some success, to other types of addictive behaviour, such as gambling, drug taking, sex and drinking alcohol. As shown in the chapter, these particular theories are also equally relevant for understanding the psychological processes at work in those who exercise to extremes.

Notes

1   Source: 'How much is too much? The development and validation of the Exercise Dependence Scale' by H. A. Hausenblas and D. Symons Downs, *Psychology and Health* (2002) vol.17, pp. 89–123. Copyright Taylor & Francis: www.tandf.co.uk/journals. Reproduced with permission.
2   Source: 'Does primary exercise dependence really exist' by D. Veale in J. Annet, B. Cripps and H. Steinberg (eds), *Exercise Addiction: Motivation for participation in sport and exercise* (1995, pp. 1–5). Copyright The British Psychological Society. Reproduced with permission.
3   Source: Copyright 1991. From *Compulsive exercise and the eating disorders* by A. Yates. Reproduced by permission of Routledge/Taylor & Francis Group, LLC.

References

Aidman, E. V. and Woollard, S. (2003) 'The influence of self-reported exercise addiction on acute emotional and physiological responses to brief exercise deprivation', *Psychology of Sport and Exercise*, 4, 225–36.

American Psychiatric Association (1994) *Diagnostic and statistical manual of mental disorders.* (4th edition), New York: American Psychiatric Association.

Annett, J., Cripps, B. and Steinberg, H. (eds) (1995) *Exercise addiction: Motivation for participation in sport and exercise*, Leicester: The British Psychological Society.

Baekeland, F. (1970) 'Exercise deprivation: Sleep and psychological reactions' *Archives of General Psychiatry*, 22, 365–9.

Bamber, D., Cockerill, I. M. and Carroll, D. (2000) 'The pathological status of exercise dependence', *British Journal of Sports Medicine*, 34, 25–132.

BBC (1990) *Fit to Drop*, BBC Television Forty Minutes series.

Blaydon, M. J., Lindner, K. J. and Kerr, J. H. (2002) 'Metamotivational characteristics of eating-disordered and exercise-dependent triathletes', *Psychology of Sport and Exercise*, 3, 223–36.

Blaydon, M. J., Lindner, K. J. and Kerr, J. H. (2004) 'Metamotivational characteristics of exercise dependence and eating disorders in highly active amateur sport participants', *Personality and Individual Differences*, 36, 1419–32.

Bramble, D. M. and Lieberman, D. E. (2004) 'Endurance running and the evolution of *Homo*', *Nature*, 432, 345–52.

Brown, R. I. F. (1993) 'Some contributions of the study of gambling to the study of other addictions', in W. R. Eadington and J. A. Cornelius (eds) *Gambling behaviour and problem gambling*, Reno NV: University of Nevada, 241–72.

Brown, R. I. F. (1997) 'A theoretical model of the behavioural addictions – applied to offending', in J. E. Hodge, M. McMurran and C. R. Hollin (eds) *Addicted to crime?*, Chichester: John Wiley, 14–65.

Chapman, C. L. and DeCastro, J. M. (1990) 'Running addiction: Measurement and associated psychological characteristics', *Journal of Sports Medicine*, 30, 283–90.

Cohen, R. (1995) 'Video interviews: "hooked" on exercise', in J. Annett, B. Cripps and H. Steinberg (eds) *Exercise addiction: Motivation for participation in sport and exercise*, Leicester: The British Psychological Society, 54–60.

Cox, R. and Orford, J. (2004) 'A qualitative study of the meaning of exercise for people who could be labelled as "addicted" to exercise – can "addiction" be applied to high frequency exercising?' *Addiction Research and Theory*, 12, 167–88.

Cripps, B. (1995) 'Exercise addiction and chronic fatigue syndrome: case study of a mountain biker', in J. Annett, B. Cripps and H. Steinberg (eds) *Exercise addiction: Motivation for participation in sport and exercise*, Leicester: The British Psychological Society, 22–33.

De Coverly Veale, D. M. W. (1987) 'Exercise dependence', *British Journal of Addiction*, 82, 735–40.

Glasser, W. (1976) *Positive addiction*, New York: Harper & Row.

Griffiths, M. (1996) 'Behavioural addiction: an issue for everybody?', *Journal of Workplace Learning*, 8, 19–25.

Griffiths, M. (1997) 'Exercise addiction: A case study', *Addiction Research*, 5, 161–8.

Griffiths, M. (2002) *Gambling, and gaming addictions in adolescence*, Leicester: British Psychological Society/Blackwells.

Guardian Unlimited (2004) 'Keep on running', 19 July. Online. Available www. guardian.co.uk.

Hausenblas, H. A. and Giacobbi, P. R. (2004) 'Relationship between exercise dependence symptoms and personality', *Personality and Individual Differences*, 36, 1265–73.

Hausenblas, H. A. and Symons Downs, D. (2002a) 'Exercise dependence: A systematic review', *Psychology of Sport and Exercise*, 3, 89–123.

Hausenblas, H. A. and Symons Downs, D. (2002b) 'How much is too much? The development and validation of the Exercise Dependence Scale', *Psychology and Health*, 17, 387–404.

Independent (2004) 'You don't have to be mad to do this. But it helps', 2 June. Online. Available http://news.independent.co.uk.

Ironman (2005) 'Ironman Triathlon World Championship', 12 January. Online. Available www.Ironmanlive.com.

Japan Times (2005) 'German jogger finishes 43-day run', 16 May, 18.

Kerr, J. H. (1997) *Motivation and emotion in sport: Reversal theory*, Hove: Psychology Press.

Keski-Rahkonen, A. (2001) 'Exercise dependence – a myth or a real issue?', *European Eating Disorders Review*, 9, 279–83.

Long, C. G., Smith, J., Midgley, M. and Cassidy, T. (1993) 'Over-exercising in anorexic and normal samples: Behaviour and attitudes', *Journal of Mental Health*, 2, 321–7.

Loumidis, K. S. and Roxborough, H. (1995) 'A cognitive-behavioural approach to excessive exercising', in J. Annett, B. Cripps and H. Steinberg (eds) *Exercise addiction: Motivation for participation in sport and exercise*, Leicester: The British Psychological Society, 45–53.

Morgan, W. P. (1979) 'Negative addiction in runners', *Physician and Sports Medicine*, 7, 57–70.

Murphy, M. H. (1994) 'Sport and drugs and runner's high', in J. Kremer and D. Scully (eds) *Psychology in sport*, London: Taylor & Francis, 173–86.

Ogden, J., Veale, D. M. W. and Summers, Z. (1997) 'The development and validation of the Exercise Dependence Questionnaire', *Addiction Research*, 5, 343–56.

Orford, J. (2001) *Excessive appetites: A psychological view of addictions* (2nd edition), Chichester: John Wiley.

Pierce, E. F. (1994) 'Exercise dependence syndrome in runners', *Sports Medicine*, 18, 149–55.

Pierce, E. F., McGowan, R. W. and Lynn, T. D. (1993) 'Exercise dependence in relation to competitive orientation in runners', *Journal of Sports Medicine and Physical Fitness*, 33, 189–94.

Robbins, J. and Joseph, P. (1985) 'Experiencing exercise withdrawal: Possible consequences of therapeutic and mastery running', *Journal of Sport Psychology*, 7, 23–39.

Run Across America (2004) Online. Available www.runacrossamerica2004.com/stage.

Sachs, M. L. and Pargman, D. (1979) 'Running addiction: A depth interview examination', *Journal of Sport Behavior*, 2, 143–55.

Seheult, C. (1995) 'Hooked on the "buzz": History of a body-building addict', in J. Annett, B. Cripps and H. Steinberg (eds) *Exercise addiction: Motivation for participation in sport and exercise*, Leicester: The British Psychological Society, 40–4.

Steinberg, H., Sykes, E. A. and LeBoutillier, N. (1995) 'Exercise addiction: Indirect measures of 'endorphins'?', in J. Annett, B. Cripps and H. Steinberg (eds) *Exercise addiction: Motivation for participation in sport and exercise*, Leicester: The British Psychological Society, 6–14.

Szabo, A. (1998) 'Studying the psychological impact of exercise deprivation: Are experimental studies hopeless?', *Journal of Sport Behavior*, 21, 139–47.

Szabo, A. (2000) 'Physical activity as a source of psychological dysfunction', in S. J. H. Biddle, K. R. Fox and S. H. Boutcher (eds) *Physical activity and psychological well-being*, London: Routledge, 130–95.

Terry, A., Szabo, A. and Griffiths, M. (2004) 'The exercise addiction inventory: A new brief screening tool', *Addiction Research and Theory*, 12, 489–99.

Thaxton, L. (1982) 'Physiological and psychological effects of short term exercise addiction on habitual runners', *Journal of Sport Psychology*, 4, 73–80.

Thompson, J. K. and Blanton, P. (1987) 'Energy conservation and exercise dependence: A sympathetic arousal hypothesis', *Medicine and Science in Sports and Exercise*, 19, 91–7.

Veale, D. (1995) 'Does primary exercise dependence really exist?', in J. Annett, B. Cripps and H. Steinberg (eds) *Exercise addiction: Motivation for participation in sport and exercise*, Leicester: The British Psychological Society, 1–5.

Weinberg, G. M. (1998) 'Motivation in ultra distance runners: A reversal theory approach to optimal experience', unpublished doctoral dissertation, Santa Barbara CA: Fielding Institute.

Whiting, H. T. A. (1994) 'Exercise addiction: Motivation for participation in sport and exercise', submission for a Satellite Professional Development Workshop, The British Psychological Society, Sport and Exercise Psychology Section.

Witman, G. W., Fuller, N. P. and Taber, J. I. (1987) 'Patterns of polyaddictions in alcoholism patients and high school students', in W. R. Eadington (ed.), *Research in gambling: Proceedings of the Seventh International Conference on gambling and risk-taking*, Reno NV: University of Nevada.

Yates, A. (1991) *Compulsive exercise and the eating disorders*, New York: Brunner Mazel.

2 A foundation for understanding

Theoretical approaches to the study of dependencies

As we have seen, Orford (2001) and Brown (1993, 1997) have proposed theoretical models to explain the psychological processes involved in forms of pathological dependencies such as drinking, gambling, and drug taking. In addition, they have extended their models to include other activities not traditionally considered to be dependencies or addictions. These include excessive exercising, eating, and sex, and form part of what Orford (2001, p. 3) called 'the core addictions'. These two behavioural addiction models have been chosen by the present authors because of their comprehensive nature, enlightened approach and the fact that they share a number of key concepts. Both have been applied to exercise addiction. This chapter will outline the basic premises of these two approaches, identify the common ground, and point out any conceptual differences between them. Illustrative examples of exercise-based research findings related to Brown's model will also be included.

Brown (e.g. 1988) extended his work to include reversal theory (Apter, 2001), and this work will also be described in this chapter. It is this combined theoretical approach that will emerge from the discussion as being the most helpful for explaining the motivation behind primary and secondary exercise dependence.

Before moving on to examine the conceptual arguments in Orford's (2001) and Brown's (1993, 1997) models, it is important to extend the discussion begun in Chapter 1 to understand why both authors have rejected the medical or disease models of dependence. In everyday thought and language, and in the study of addictions or dependencies in psychology, ideas of chemical dependency and substance abuse have tended to dominate thinking and have diverted attention from other types of dependencies. As Brown (1997) stated:

> the popular belief is that addictions are diseases which cause addicts to lose all control over the taking of a substance. Or that just taking even one dose of it (in the case of heroin) can produce irreversible physical effects on body tissue so that the addict will need more and more of it for the rest of their life. The most common allied belief is that total

abstinence and constant dependence on AA groups, doctors, or Jesus groups is then for ever necessary to avoid being overwhelmed by the craving and by the urges to take the substance again in the same destructive way.

(Brown, 1997, p. 14–15)

Brown (1997) argued that this type of model is only useful in explaining those addictions where substances are sucked, swallowed, breathed or injected, and useless in explaining other types of addiction such as gambling or excessive sex. Orford (2001, p. 2; see also Chapter 1) expressed similar sentiments and also made a case for changing the shape of the field of addictions. He accepted that addictions could resemble diseases if they became very strong, but, like Brown (1997), he felt that the analogy was not a useful one because there were also many ways in which addictions did not resemble a physical disease. However, Orford (2001) was also quick to point out that although his model was not biologically based:

This is not to deny the probable contribution of genetic determinants at many points in developing and giving up addictions – to totally discount such influence would be to fly in the face of all we know about the complex interaction of genes and the environment in the determination of all human behaviour. But although biology comes into the picture in many places – in the psychopharmacological effects of drugs for example, in brain systems that may underlie reward, in secondary neuroadaption processes, or in the effects of strong appetitive attachments upon mental and physical ill-health – the present model is in essence a psychological one.

(Orford, 2001, p. 344)

In Brown's (1997) model as well, the major factors in the development of and recovery from addictions are psychological 'although physical processes are seen as providing strong secondary support' (Brown, 1997, p. 17). Thus, both authors are in favour of broadening the concept of dependencies and, as will be shown, putting a greater emphasis on the subjective experience of the individuals concerned.

The following sections summarize the main points of Orford's (2001) Social-Behavioural-Cognitive-Moral Model of Excessive Appetites and Brown's (1993, 1997) Hedonic Management Model of Addictions.

The Social-Behavioural-Cognitive-Moral Model of Excessive Appetites

As mentioned in Chapter 1, Orford (2001) preferred the term 'excessive appetite' to 'addiction' but used the two terms interchangeably. Here is a reminder of how he defined his understanding of the two terms:

> An addiction, or an 'excessive appetite' to be more precise, is the same whether its object is alcohol, gambling, heroin, tobacco, eating or sex. It is best thought of as an over-attachment to a drug, object or activity and the process of overcoming it is largely a naturally occurring one.
>
> (Orford, 2001, p. xi)

This view of excessive appetites is fundamental to his whole model. Orford's (2001) model, a summary of which is shown in Figure 2.1, consists of eight basic arguments (Orford, 2001, pp. 341–4), which are précised in the paragraphs that follow.

Orford's interest, research and publications have focused on excessive drinking and its effects on the family and local community in a number of countries (e.g. Orford, 1992; Orford *et al.*, 1998; Orford and Velleman, 1990). In his model, he has identified a range of appetitive activities that, when taken to excess, have a profound effect on the quality of life of the individuals who participate in them (e.g. drinking alcohol, gambling, hard and soft drug use, binge eating, sex and exercising). As family and social life are also usually affected, family and friends are likely to become concerned about the behaviour. Excessive appetitive activities are also likely to be costly to communities as systems are set up to provide mutual and expert help and treatment to deal with them.

A person's involvement in excessive appetitive activities is brought about by a number of factors that interact. According to Orford, these factors, which can act as incentives or disincentives, include personality, opportunities to take part in the activity and the normative influence of friends. It is thought that these activities can be beneficial to the individual in, for example, modulating moods, enhancing self-identity and facilitating different forms of self-expression. Some of the strongest determinants of excessive appetitive activities are ecological, socio-economic or cultural. Understanding how the same activities are interpreted and how they become excessive can be assisted by taking cross-cultural and long-term historical perspectives.

Orford argued that appetitive behaviours involve dynamic changing processes over time. Within these processes, changes in behaviour are caused by a mix of attitudes, experiences, values and activities, and they are likely to intensify according to the law of proportionate effect when incentives are comparatively strong and restraints are comparatively weak. At different stages of change, the same activity may provide different personal functions for any one person, and transitions between stages may be predicted by different personal and social factors.

Orford utilized learning theory to explain the psychological processes involved in the development of excessive appetites:

> The combination of positive incentive, operant learning, based on mood modification and other positive rewards from activity, plus negative

reinforcement, 'coping' functions of activity, in combination with the establishment of associations between multiple cues and the appetitive activity, plus the abundant opportunities that exist for the development of behaviour-enhancing expectancies, attributions, images and fantasies, provides *a powerful set of processes for the development of a strong attachment.*

(Orford, 2001, pp. 342–3)

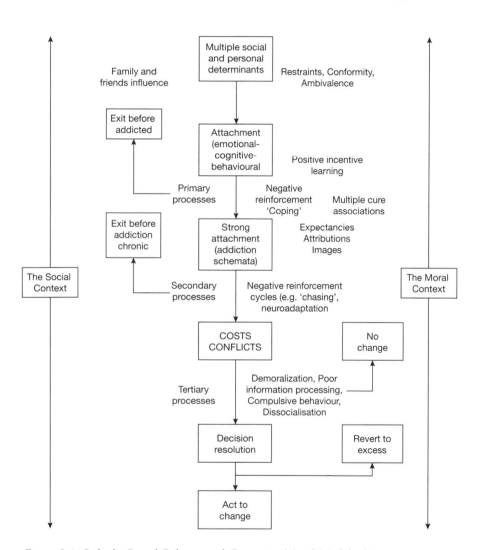

Figure 2.1 Orford's Social-Behavioural-Cognitive-Moral Model of Excessive Appetites

Source: *Excessive appetites: A view of psychological addictions* by J. Orford (2001). Copyright John Wiley & Sons Limited. Reproduced with permission.

Orford (2001, p. 343) identified the formation of what are referred to as 'secondary emotional cycles' (e.g. chasing losses in gambling and secrecy in most activities) and how they become important in the new, acquired motivation associated with the development of a strong appetite for a particular activity. A number of changes take place, so that the activity becomes increasingly salient and is no longer moderated by personal perceptions or judgments that previously kept the behaviour within certain bounds. Recollections, thoughts and attention schemata are frequently induced as the person becomes preoccupied by the activity. The activity now provides a wider range of functions for the individual, some of which are seen as serving non-social purposes and which may become automatic and functionally autonomous.

Factors such as age, sex, personal values, social roles and circumstances govern the increased risk of incurring costs (physical, social, immediate or long term, affecting self or others) from appetitive behaviour. Strong attachments to appetitive behaviour are personally and socially defined and likely to be characterized by ambivalence and, as costs accrue, may well result in a conflict of motives. These are likely to become more obvious and personally disturbing to the individual (e.g. demoralization, poor information processing, compulsive behaviour, changes in social role and group) and they further strengthen the process of addiction:

> Furthermore, at the very core of addiction, according to this view, is not so much attachment per se but rather conflict about attachment. The restraints, controls and disincentives that create conflict out of attachment are personally, socially and culturally relative.
>
> (Orford, 2001, p. 347)

Orford was convinced that many people cut down or stop excessive appetitive behaviour on their own, without help from experts. What is more, reversion rates to the activity after treatment or other attempts to change are high and show similar relapse patterns across different excessive appetitive behaviours. He argued that a wide range of treatments based on expert help are only modestly successful and may be operating under a set of common fundamental change processes. Orford thought that the change process had both cognitive (a decision or resolution to change) and action or behavioural elements and was the natural outcome of the conflict that is associated with the gathering costs that accompany the excessive appetitive behaviour. Social and spiritual processes can play a role in the change processes, whether they are individually driven or expert-assisted.

The Hedonic Management Model of Addictions

The roots of Brown's (1997) model can be found in his research work on gambling and his work on other addictions (e.g. Anderson and Brown,

1984; Brown, 1986, 1987, 1989). Brown (1997) set out his Hedonic Management Model of Addictions, which is based on cognitive social-learning theory, in twelve propositions. The first seven deal with how addictions develop and become established, and the next three deal with recovery and relapse. The last two are statements about: (a) the need to distinguish addictions from habits, obsessions, compulsions, or attachments; and (b) the need to recognize addictions as value free and having both valuable and undesirable consequences. The key elements of Brown's (1997) propositions, represented graphically in Figure 2.2, will be outlined in the next section.

Brown claimed that people learn how to maintain good hedonic tone (the subjective experience of mood and emotional state as pleasurable) for as much of the time as possible by manipulating their experience of arousal, mood and well-being. This manipulation provides the opportunity to plan ongoing events and activities to be rewarding, thus maintaining high levels of hedonic tone and allowing people to keep on enjoying life in general. If regularly reproduced, some pleasant states may come to act as secondary goals or drives. With regard to modulating arousal, he referred to Apter (1982), who has identified a number of common techniques for raising or lowering arousal.

The concept of arousal utilized by psychologists such as Brown (1997), Thayer (1989) and Apter (1982) is psychological or phenomenological rather than physiological in nature. Engaging in any form of physical work or exercise involves increased breathing and heart rates and other related cardiovascular biological processes. All of these contribute to increased physiological activation or arousal levels. The psychological concept of arousal, although thought to be linked to physiological arousal, is concerned with an individual's subjective experience and interpretation of his or her own levels of arousal, and different levels of arousal can relate to different levels of hedonic tone (e.g. high arousal can be experienced as either anxiety or excitement). It is this concept of arousal that is used in this book.

Brown pointed out that people vary in their vulnerabilities to addictions and that the individual's predisposing vulnerabilities either (a) increase a person's 'hedonic gap' (i.e. the discrepancy between the levels of dysphoria or negative feeling states [e.g. anxiety, restlessness, depression] they can tolerate and those they habitually experience; the greater the hedonic gap, the greater their vulnerability) or (b) reduce the range of easily accessible rewarding activities (Brown, 1997, pp. 24–6).

Brown argued that the actual initiation of an addiction may develop gradually over a period of time or occur suddenly, as in his example (Brown, 1997) of the person with chronic low arousal who goes gambling and has a big win at the first attempt. Here the massive increase in pleasant arousal and euphoria will be enough to relieve feelings of dysphoria (perhaps long-term) and dramatically alter that person's preferences for the various activities easily accessible to them. Alternatively, the initiation of an addiction may take longer, gradually drawing a person into a rewarding pattern of activity.

1. **Management of hedonic tone**
    Individual learns to manipulate arousal, mood, and experiences to sustain pleasant hedonic tone.

2. **Vulnerabilities**
    Personal vulnerability to addiction increases hedonic gap and decreases number of easily accessible rewarding activities.

3. **Initiation**
    Gradual or sudden discovery of an activity which is a powerful and effective means of manipulating hedonic tone.

4. **Addictive activity choice**
    Choice depends on range of activities available; social support; inherent properties for affecting hedonic tone through e.g. changes in arousal; developed skills for use of an activity in hedonic tone manipulation.

5. **Development of acquired drive and increasing salience**
    Addiction results from a positive feedback loop involving cognitive failures and development of an acquired drive towards the goal of pleasant feeling states with a single activity increasingly salient as source of reward.

6. **Cycles**
    Engagement in addictive activity comes in repeated cycles which make up a serial. Build-up of conditioning effects and reinforcement, rituals and cognitive distortion of belief systems occurs.

7. **Established addiction**
    A single addictive activity fully developed as a motivational monopoly dominating thinking and behaviour. Decisions made solely on basis of extremely short-term reward and avoidance of withdrawal symptoms.

Figure 2.2 A summary of the first seven 'propositions' or stages of Brown's (1997) Hedonic Management Model of Addiction

The person then becomes increasingly dependent on that activity for his or her everyday management of hedonic tone, thus also changing his or her preference for other accessible activities. In either case, the activity becomes a powerful and effective means of manipulating hedonic tone with the aim of sustaining long periods of euphoria or providing relief from dysphoria.

According to Brown (1997), choosing a particular addictive activity or substance depends on at least four factors. One of the most important is how efficiently a person learns to use an activity or substance to maintain high positive hedonic tone. This occurs through modulation of a person's naturally occurring patterns of arousal and subjective experience as part of an acquired drive. The learning process and the development of skills with which to manipulate hedonic tone usually take time, unless a person discovers the benefits by chance. The power of the intrinsic properties of an activity to affect a person's arousal levels and hedonic tone is a second important factor, along with the range of possible activities available to a person and the degree of social support for an activity. Brown indicated that activities such as smoking and drinking, and many of the other addictive substances and activities, are bi-directional. This means that they can be used both to increase or decrease arousal depending on how a person uses them, and many of those who become skilled in the use of one bi-directional technique often stick with it and have no need to learn any other. However, Brown also noted that others seem to continually try new substances, activities, and techniques, and this may explain the development of poly-addictions or cross-addictions and the use of combined activities such as drinking and gambling. The stronger the reinforcement effects the faster the development of an addiction (e.g. for exercise, relatively slow and subtle; for cocaine use, immediate and powerful). Brown also pointed out that the physical properties of a few substances produce steeper tolerance gradients, but they lead to the same effect. 'However, in general it is not the choice of substance or activity which is so important as the ways in which it is used' (Brown, 1997, p. 28).

In the Hedonic Management Model, addictions are thought to become established as the result of a series of cognitive failures (e.g. poor planning and decision-making) and the development of emotional and cognitive positive feedback loops. In turn, these lead to an acquired drive for particular feeling states as goals. In this process, a single activity becomes increasingly salient. In Brown's opinion, this increasing salience comes about through a person's poor self-awareness or vigilance, inadequate short-term planning and crisis management, and faulty decision-making. In addition to a person's own inner conflict about the addictive behaviour, conflict arises as others notice and become concerned about it, and the person's range of easily accessible rewarding activities becomes limited. As salience increases, so too do the tolerance levels, withdrawals and relief action that lead to salience being increased even more. All this, Brown hypothesizes, contributes to the further conditioning of the addictive process:

> the addictive behaviour acquires a salience and begins to produce its own consequent life-problems (its 'alcohol-related problems', its severe consequences of excessive gambling) which serve to make the further manipulation of hedonic tone even *more* necessary and rewarding.
>
> (Brown, 1997, p. 36)

Brown has argued that, during the later stages of their development, addictions come in repeated 'cycles' or 'episodes' where, for example, an episode for an alcoholic might be a single night's drinking or a much longer binge that could last several weeks. Such episodes begin with biased anticipation of how easy it will be to achieve and maintain pleasant hedonic experience and how intense an experience it will be. In the middle stages, addictions are characterized by a total focus on the present, and addicts will often try to boost their pleasant state (e.g. by betting more heavily during gambling episodes). If episodes take place often enough, they develop into a 'serial':

> During the later stages of its development the engagement in addictive activity comes in repeated cycles or in episodes which make up a serial, during which there is a build-up of: (i) potent classical conditioning effects and schedules of reinforcement; (ii) rituals inducing the sought-after feeling states; (iii) dysfunctional cognitive distortions and belief systems; and, possibly, (iv) routines facilitating entry to partially or wholly dissociated states.
>
> (Brown, 1997, p. 41)

Once the addiction becomes fully established, a single addictive activity has such salience that it has the power to control a person's thinking, feeling and behaviour in a motivational monopoly that makes it almost the only source of reward in the continuous maintenance of high hedonic tone. It produces mounting conflict, and personal decision-making is then based on achieving extremely short-term reward or relief and avoiding withdrawals, as simple crisis management. Salience, conflict, relief, low self-esteem, and relapse and reinstatement, all classic psychological elements in addictions, are now apparent.

For the person with an addiction, reduction or extinction of the addictive activity involves improving his or her self-awareness, vigilance and decision-making as well as becoming more tolerant of short-term unpleasant feelings or negative hedonic tone. Improvements in hedonic tone require better planning for its medium- and long-term manipulation through the re-establishment of a much wider range of rewarding activities and easily attainable rewarding experiences, thus achieving 'a wider dispersal of sources of reward and an improved overall rate of reward or quality of life' (Brown, 1997, p. 46). The more successful the person is in planning and the process of dispersal, the less the chance of relapse to the previous levels of addictive activity and the lower his or her vulnerability to cross-addictions.

Similarities and differences between Brown's and Orford's models

Both models challenge the medical or disease model of addictions, but both agree that there is a probable link to biological processes. These two behavioural theories share a good deal of common conceptual ground. For example, both Brown's and Orford's models emphasize the subjective nature of addictions and stress the importance of the processes by which activities may become salient. They also both describe how tolerance and withdrawal symptoms play a role and emphasize the importance of negative consequences and especially conflict in family and social life. In addition, both models outline how people become totally absorbed by the activity so that work, study or everyday tasks are severely disrupted. The two models also stress the influence of operant learning, feedback loops and reinforcement processes, poor vigilance, planning and decision-making (Brown, 1997) and information processing (Orford, 2001). Finally, both models have proposed the strong possibility of relapse or reversion at any time after the addictive activity has apparently ceased.

However, there are also some differences between the two models. The key differences include: the importance of mood modulation; the import-ance given to cultural and moral versus value-free dimensions; and the relative importance or unimportance of expert counselling in the treatment of addictions. Brown placed a much stronger emphasis on arousal and the manipulation of hedonic tone in addictive activity than Orford. Orford did include the notion of mood modification and emotional regulation, but it is not the central focus of his model in the same way that it is in Brown's model.

Orford stressed the importance of cultural and moral influences on addictions, while Brown's model barely mentions cultural influences and is free of any moral overtones. Orford considered that the spiritual and moral dimensions could assist people in giving up excess and retained a moral dimension in his model; Brown, however, was keen to cast any suggestion of moral judgment aside. He claimed that moral models tend to interpret addictive behaviours as bad, reflecting personal weakness or even wickedness and evil and requiring punishment and deterrence, if not evangelical conversion or spiritual regeneration, in order to be cured. He wanted a value-free concept of addiction, arguing that: 'Clearly not even the most destructive addiction at the furthest end of the good–bad value scale is always entirely an unmixed disaster' (Brown, 1997, pp. 50–1). The twelfth and final proposition of his Hedonic Management Model of Addictions concerns the importance of a value-free concept of addictions.

Orford was somewhat dismissive of expert help and argued that change towards moderation or abstinence was a natural outcome in the history of the development of a strongly appetitive activity. Brown, however, did envisage a role for counselling and intervention where it could help the addict deal with the accumulating health, social, legal, and relationship problems arising from the addictive activity. Also, Brown thought counselling could play a part in helping addicts to improve self-awareness and assist them to realize the extent of the addictive activity's salience and how feedback loops work to reinforce the activity. He considered this to be necessary to bring about complete changes in the management of hedonic tone during recovery, as well as further in the future, in trying to prevent reversions and relapses.

Brown's model was selected as the preferred option for providing a meaningful theoretical foundation for understanding exercise addiction. Brown's explanations of the role that changes in arousal play in the addictive process were intuitively appealing to the authors, and thought to be especially relevant when exercise addiction was under scrutiny. In contrast, Orford gave little emphasis to arousal in his model. Another reason for choosing Brown's approach was his perceptive and skilful use of reversal theory to augment his arguments, adding to his explanations of how addicted individuals manipulate their arousal levels and hedonic tone. The next section examines how Brown's (1993, 1997) model was applied in a research study of excessive exercise. The results of this study provide strong support for the various theoretical propositions in Brown's (1993, 1997) model.

Applying Brown's (1997) model to exercise addiction

Griffiths (e.g. Griffiths and Cooper, 2003; Griffiths *et al.*, 2004; Griffiths and Wood, 2001) has carried out research into gaming, gambling and other excessive behaviours and has built Brown's (1997) model of addiction into some of his research. This research included a study of exercise addiction where an excessive exerciser's behaviour was examined using Brown's (1997) model (Griffiths, 1997). He described a case study of 25-year-old 'Joanna', a very good amateur Jiu-Jitsu athlete, who began taking part in the sport in her late teens. She came from a stable background, had good high school qualifications, ate very well and described herself as being in excellent physical condition (except for an arm injury that had occurred during a recent Jiu-Jitsu session). She had never taken anabolic steroids. She did not think of herself as being addicted, but recognized that she did have a problem surrounding exercise.

In reviewing the evidence, Griffiths (1997) was convinced that exercise had taken over Joanna's life. The time that she spent exercising had increased considerably over the previous five years, and she experienced 'highs' in connection with different aspects of her exercising and withdrawal symptoms when she could not exercise. She also experienced conflict over her excessive exercise behaviour, which had resulted in the loss of friends, the breakdown of her personal relationship, poorer academic work and considerable debt. Furthermore, she continued training despite injury and the risk of permanent damage, against medical advice. As is shown below, Joanna's exercise behaviour fulfilled Brown's (1993) key components of addiction. Griffiths' (1997) somewhat lengthy, but valuable account is included here:

> *Salience:* Jiu-Jitsu is the most important activity in Joanna's life above everything else. Even when not actually engaged in the activity she will

be thinking about the next training session or competition. She estimates that she spends approximately six hours a day (and sometimes more) involved in training (e.g. weight training, jogging, general exercise etc.).

Last year she even walked out of one of her finals papers to attend a Jiu-Jitsu competition in another part of the country (i.e. she had a train to catch so she left early). She got behind with her coursework due to exercise because she claimed she could not find the time to study. She likes to exercise both in the morning and evening but if she misses a morning session she has an extra long evening session to make up for it. Further to this, she has started to go swimming during her lunch hour.

Tolerance: Joanna started Jiu-Jitsu at an evening class once a week in her mid-teens and built up slowly over a period of about five years. She now exercises every single day and the lengths of the sessions are getting longer and longer which suggests she has become tolerant to the activity. When she cannot actually engage in Jiu-Jitsu she has to do some other form of exercise. This perhaps could be argued to be a kind of cross-tolerance.

Withdrawal: Joanna claims she gets highly agitated and irritable if she is unable to exercise. When her arm was bandaged up because of an arm injury she went for three hour jogs instead. She claims she also gets headaches and feels nauseous if she goes for more than a day without training or has to miss a scheduled session.

Euphoria: Joanna experiences euphoria in a number of ways. She feels very high if she has done well in a Jiu-Jitsu competition and when she wins she gets the biggest buzz of all. She also feels high if she's trained hard and for a long time. She is only productive in other areas of her life (re: academic work) if her exercise has been completed (i.e. she can only function normally after exercise). She claims she often trains until late at night and then works on essays or reports through the night. At times like this she claims she feels like she 'is on speed' and keeps on working until she feels the need to exercise again.

Conflict: Joanna's relationship with her long-term partner has finished as a result of her exercise. She claims she never spent much time with him and says she is not even bothered about their break-up. She claims she has become 'a bit of a loner' with few friends as a result of her excessive exercising. Added to this her degree suffered because of the lack of time and concentration. She also freely acknowledges that she is spending too much time engaged in exercise and knows she should be doing more important things in her life.

Loss of control: Joanna claims she cannot stop herself engaging in exercise when she 'gets the urge'. Once started she has to do a minimum of a few hours exercise. She claims she has a total lack of concentration during lectures. She also claims she has an inability to revise unless she has done her exercise.

Relapse: Joanna can only go a few days of no exercise before her day-to-day living becomes absolutely unbearable. If she misses a competition she is just as bad. The thought that she could have won a medal but was not there is particularly painful for her. She has continually tried to stop and/or cut down but claims she cannot. She becomes highly anxious if she is unable to engage in exercise and then has to go out and train to make herself feel better. She is well aware that exercise has taken over her life but feels powerless to stop it.

Negative consequences: Joanna spends money beyond her means to maintain her exercising habit (e.g. on entrance fees for weight training, swimming etc.). She also spends a lot of time between two towns and therefore she has a lot of dual memberships of various leisure clubs. She is financially in debt not just because she is a student but also because she funds herself to get to Jiu-Jitsu competitions up and down the country. She claims she resorted to (unspecified) socially unacceptable means in order to get money to fund herself. She also misses many lectures to go and exercise instead because there is no one telling her she cannot do it. She is now particularly worried about her injured arm which is never given enough time to heal properly before Joanna gets the urge to take part in Jiu-Jitsu training and competitions. Her doctor has advised her to give up the sport because he thinks she will do permanent damage to her arm. This is something she feels she is totally unable to do even if it means permanent damage.

(Griffiths, 1997, pp. 163–4)[1]

In a final set of comments, Griffiths (1997) pointed out that Joanna had recently been to a doctor and been prescribed minor tranquillizers to help calm her nerves when not exercising. She had reduced her Jiu-Jitsu and other exercise activities and could function 'normally'. Griffiths (1997), however, was uncertain about what would happen when she stopped taking the tranquillizers.

Griffiths (1997) used Brown's (1993) model to good effect, showing how the model was relevant for understanding exercise addiction. An additional strength of Brown's (1997) theoretical thinking is the way in which he linked his model to reversal theory (Apter, 1982, 2001).

Extensions of Brown's (1993, 1997) work to include reversal theory

Brown (1997) deserves credit for his efforts to change thinking in the field of addictions. However, as he pointed out (Brown, 2001), attempting to change the consensus was not an easy task. Although his first publication on reversal theory, subjective experience, and addiction and relapse was published in the late 1980s (Brown, 1988), and although his model was 'inspired by reversal theory' (Brown, 2001, p. 161), Brown kept this aspect somewhat removed from the general thrust of his Hedonic Management Model of Addictions. He felt that there were already enough problems with getting his model accepted, without the added complications of reversal theory:

> Unfortunately the full sophistication that reversal theory could bring to this new general theory of addiction could seldom be presented. This is because it was difficult enough for the normally cognitive-behavioral and empirically oriented audience or readership of psychologists to absorb a new theory of addictive activities without also requiring them to absorb an equally new and, to them, even stranger new theory of reversals in the same operation.
>
> (Brown, 2001, p. 163)

Of course, both the Hedonic Management Model of Addictions and reversal theory can stand on their own as independent theoretical approaches, but it is their use in combination that provides added power and sophistication to the understanding of addictions. Brown (1997), with considerable insight, has explained how the addiction process works, and the role of motivation and subjective experience within it. On a step-by-step basis, he has laid his twelve basic propositions down on the table in a manner akin to a winning hand in cards. What reversal theory brings to this table is a new way of reading the 'cards' of human behaviour. The theory adds an additional level to the analysis of addictive activities by introducing the metamotivational level or dimension to understanding the complexity, changeability, and variety of human behaviour, including addictive behaviour. It is at this point that readers who are unfamiliar with reversal theory are directed to Appendix A, which outlines the main concepts of reversal theory in sufficient detail for comprehending how the theory is applied in this book. Those readers who may want to read more fully about reversal theory are directed to the main reversal theory texts (Apter, 1982, 1989/2006, 2001).

Exactly how reversal theory adds to the understanding of aspects of addictive behaviour in Brown's model can be illustrated by examples from Brown's work on gambling addiction, which are equally applicable to other forms of potentially addictive pursuits and addiction in general.

How reversal theory can enhance aspects of Brown's (1997) model

In his first theoretical proposition, Brown (1997) has emphasized the importance of arousal in the addictive process and how a person learns to manipulate arousal patterns to maintain high positive hedonic tone. In reversal theory, the serious (telic) and playful (paratelic) states have a special relationship with a person's experience of arousal levels (felt arousal). In the serious (telic) state, high levels are usually experienced as unpleasant (anxiety), and low levels of arousal are usually preferred and experienced as pleasant (relaxation); in the playful (paratelic) state, high arousal is usually preferred and experienced as pleasant (excitement) and low arousal as unpleasant (boredom). Brown (1988) outlined how this relationship could help a person to manipulate arousal in a gambling situation. For example, on arriving at a casino or other gambling facility a person might be in the playful (paratelic) state, but experiencing low arousal as boredom. The person's expectations or the environmental cues (the general atmosphere, brightly coloured lights and glitzy décor; uncertainty, risk taking; and the familiar sights and sounds of gambling) might serve to increase arousal levels and allow the person to experience excitement. Here the person has manipulated his or her arousal level by deliberately going to the gambling location. In another scenario, a person might be experiencing high arousal and anxiety in the serious (telic) state on arrival at a gambling establish-ment. In this state, similar environmental cues could trigger a reversal to the playful (paratelic) state. In this state the person can then re-interpret the existing high arousal and experience it as excitement. In the second case, the gambling location was used as a means of inducing a reversal so that high arousal could be experienced as pleasant; in the first case, the same location was used as a means to increase arousal from low to high levels. In both cases the pay-off was improved positive hedonic tone and the individuals concerned had learned how to achieve it. Achieving and maintaining these desirable feeling states for as long as possible can become goals in themselves (Brown, 2001). Other characteristics of the gambling environment, such as strict rules, familiarity and security, provide a safe context for uncertainty and risk taking, enabling a person to experience risk through a paratelic protective frame (see Appendix A) where high arousal can be interpreted as excitement (Brown, 2001).

As Brown (1988) suggested, during gambling, psychological reversals may play a role in a person's experience of winning and losing. For example, the ordinary or normal gambler would be expected to reverse back and forth between serious and playful states when winning or losing. On the one hand, a person may be in the serious (telic) state with the goal of winning a specific sum of money. Once that person has won more than that particular sum of money, he or she may set it aside and go on playing for fun, having reversed to the playful (paratelic) state. On the other hand, a person may start to play in the playful (paratelic) state for the excitement of the action itself, but then start losing more money than intended and this may prompt a reversal to the serious (telic) state in an attempt to recoup losses.

However, according to Brown (1988), it is more likely that gambling episodes will begin when the gambler is in the playful (paratelic) state. This is because failure to win in the telic state and increasing losses will result in anxiety and unpleasant hedonic tone, and the normal gambler will be likely to cease the gambling activity relatively quickly. This idea is supported by Anderson and Brown's (1984) research findings, which suggested that normal gamblers were in the serious (telic) state when losing and the playful (paratelic) state when winning.

Brown (1988) pointed out that the metamotivational experience of addicted gamblers is likely to be different. They often enter gambling premises to recoup previous losses; they are likely to be in the telic state, experiencing high anxiety and unpleasant hedonic tone. If they eventually win, the emotional reward in the form of a sudden positive surge in hedonic tone can be highly reinforcing:

> Through learning from experience, the high arousal associated with losing may come to be seen by the most regular gamblers as potentially very strongly reinforcing. For example, if a losing gambler was to play on in a telic state and win, then the subsequent reversal in state would mean that the residual very high arousal from the telic state (where this is felt as anxiety) would be reinterpreted in the new paratelic state as excitement and become proportionately reinforcing. Thus, the content of the telic state arising from losing may well have getting the lost money back as its primary goal, but with the added learned expectation that arousal currently endured as highly unpleasant can suddenly be transformed to be experienced as pleasant excitement, resulting in an unusually intense experiential reward.
>
> (Brown, 1988, p. 197)

For the addicted gambler, the anticipation of the psychological reward associated with winning becomes increasingly salient and eventually becomes the sole source of reward as described in the fifth proposition of Brown's (1997) model. Brown (1988) argued that this is consistent with the high degree of persistence often associated with pathological gamblers in spite of very high anxiety and financial difficulties.

Brown's work showed how reversal theory can add some finer detail to the nuts and bolts of how arousal patterns can be modulated to maintain high positive hedonic tone. Although Brown's (1988) theorizing focused on the serious (telic) and playful (paratelic) states, it is probable that the other pairs of metamotivational states play an important role in a gambler's experience. For example, negativism and conformity are also associated with the experience of felt arousal and the emotions involved. Also, the transactional states, especially the autic and mastery states, have been shown to be involved in the subjective experience of winning and losing (Wilson and Kerr, 1999). More recently, new measures have been developed to allow all eight metamotivational categories to be measured; they have yet to be used in gambling research.

Around the same time that Brown was becoming interested in reversal theory, Miller (1985), the US psychologist who is well respected for his work on addictions, also recognized the potential of the theory in a publication that outlined several ways in which reversal theory could add to explanations of addictions. Miller (1985) was quite clear about the potential that reversal theory had to offer the field of addictions:

> Just a decade ago, most professionals perceived relatively little similarity among alcoholism, obesity, smoking, and drug abuse ... Recent discussions have begun to include other behavior problems within the realm of addictive behaviors: pathological gambling, certain compulsions, sexual deviations. If the theory of psychological reversals is correct, it points to a common mechanism underlying these and other pathologies, namely, dysfunctions in the reversal process. It is fascinating that the very types of psychopathology to which reversal theory is most readily applicable are also those with which we seem to have made least headway in developing successful models of etiology and treatment to date.
>
> (Miller, 1985, p. 179)

Miller (1985) recognized that dysfunctions in the reversal process could be at the root of the addictive process and that studying them might lead to improved understanding of the nature and causes of addictive behaviour. He identified four possible types of reversal pathology: (a) a very low threshold for reversal in at least one direction in a pair of states (excessive lability); (b) a high threshold for reversal in one or both directions in a pair of states (rigidity); (c) an unhealthy preponderance of one state over the other (imbalance); and (d) reliance on an addictive behaviour to bring about a reversal. As Brown (2001) pointed out, Murgatroyd and Apter (1984, 1986) (probably unknown to Miller at that time) were already exploring these and other reversal problems in some detail, and showing how they could lead to pathological behaviour. However, these early publications were geared towards counselling and psychotherapy and using the reversal theory framework as a guide to helping people change their motivation and behaviour.

Closing comments

It was not the purpose of this one short chapter to review the many competing theories and models of addiction that have come to prominence in recent years. Orford (2001) has done a much better job of doing that than the present authors could ever achieve. The task here was to identify and summarize the main concepts from what were considered to be the most relevant and serviceable theoretical explanations of addictive behaviours, including excessive exercising. Orford's and Brown's theoretical models fulfilled these requirements, but Brown's model was considered advantageous for understanding exercise addiction.

In response to the questions 'What is an addiction?' and 'What precisely is the person addicted to?', Orford's (2001) definition, that an addiction or excessive appetite is an over-attachment to a drug, object or activity, might be offered. In the present context, the activity is exercise and the focus is therefore exercise addiction or dependence. However, is this definition strictly correct? Based on Brown's (1997) arguments, it can be said that it is the pursuit of optimum hedonic tone, or 'happiness', that people are addicted to and exercise, like drinking alcohol or smoking tobacco, is just a means to that end. In addition, Brown's (1997) Hedonic Management Model explains clearly, through seven developmental stages, what causes addictions, including exercise addiction, and how they develop and become established. Both Orford (2001) and Brown (1997) are agreed that exercise is no different to other core addictions involving alcohol, gambling, heroin, tobacco, eating or sex. In examining exercise, or any of the other addictions, reversal theory adds an extra layer of understanding to how individuals optimize hedonic tone by providing a structured framework and a rational mechanism for explaining the changes in motivation involved.

Brown (1993, 1997) especially emphasized the role of hedonic management in addictive behaviour. The following chapter examines the available research evidence on the beneficial psychological effects of exercise. If Brown (1993, 1997) is correct, the results should indicate that arousal modulation, mood enhancement and emotional change are possible outcomes of taking part in exercise.

Notes

1   Source: 'Exercise addiction: A case study' by Mark Griffiths from *Addiction Research and Theory* (1997) vol. 5, pp. 161–8. Copyright Taylor & Francis Ltd: www.tandf.co.uk/journals. Reprinted by permission of the publisher.

References

Anderson, G. and Brown, R. I. F. (1984) 'Real and laboratory gambling, sensation seeking and arousal', *British Journal of Psychology*, 75, 401–10.

Apter, M. J. (1982) *The experience of motivation*, London: Academic Press.

Apter, M. J. (1989) *Reversal theory: Motivation, emotion and personality*, London: Routledge. (2nd edition published 2006.)

Apter, M. J. (ed.) (2001) *Motivational styles in everyday life: A guide to reversal theory*, Washington DC: American Psychological Association.

Apter, M. J. (2006) *Reversal theory: The dynamics of motivation, emotion and personality*, 2nd edition, Oxford: Oneworld Publications.

Brown, R. I. F. (1986) 'Arousal and sensation seeking components in the general explanation of gambling and gambling addictions', *International Journal of Addictions*, 21, 1001–16.

Brown, R. I. F. (1987) 'Pathological gambling and associated patterns of crime: Comparisons with alcohol and other drug addictions', *Journal of Gambling Behavior*, 3, 98–114.

Brown, R. I. F. (1988) 'Reversal theory and subjective experience in the explanation of addiction and relapse', in M. J. Apter, J. H. Kerr and M. P. Cowles (eds) *Progress in reversal theory*, Amsterdam: Elsevier, 191–212.

Brown, R. I. F. (1989) 'Relapses from a gambling perspective', in M. Glossop (ed.) *Relapse and addictive behaviour*, London: Croom Helm.

Brown, R. I. F. (1993) 'Some contributions of the study of gambling to the study of other addictions', in W. R. Eadington and J. A. Cornelius (eds) *Gambling behaviour and problem gambling*, Reno NV: University of Nevada, 241–72.

Brown, R. I. F. (1997) 'A theoretical model of behavioural addictions – Applied to offending', in J. E. Hodge, M. McMurran and C. R. Hollin (eds) *Addicted to crime?*, New York: Wiley, 13–65.

Brown, R. I. F. (2001) 'Addictions', in M. J. Apter (ed.) *Motivational styles in everyday life: A guide to reversal theory*, Washington DC: American Psychological Association, 155–65.

Griffiths, M. (1997) 'Exercise addiction: A case study', *Addiction Research and Theory*, 5, 161–8.

Griffiths, M. D. and Cooper, G. (2003) 'Online therapy: Implications for problem gamblers and clinicians', *British Journal of Guidance and Counselling*, 13, 113–35.

Griffiths, M. D. and Wood, R. T. A. (2001) 'The psychology of lottery gambling', *International Gambling Studies*, 1, 27–44.

Griffiths, M. D., Davies, M. N. O. and Chappell, D. (2004) 'Online computer gaming: A comparison of adolescent and adult gamers', *Journal of Adolescence*, 27, 87–96.

Miller, W. R. (1985) 'Addictive behaviour and the theory of psychological reversals', *Addictive Behaviors*, 10, 177–80.

Murgatroyd, S. and Apter, M. J. (1984) 'Eclectic psychotherapy: A structural phenomenological approach', in W. R. Dryden (ed.) *Individual psychotherapy in Britain*, London: Harper & Row, 389–414.

Murgatroyd, S. and Apter, M. J. (1986) 'A structural-phenomenological approach to eclectic psychotherapy', in J. Norcross (ed.) *Casebook of eclectic psychotherapy*, New York: Bruner/Mazel, 260–80.

Orford, J. (2001) *Excessive appetites: A psychological view of addictions*, Chichester: John Wiley.

Orford, J. (1992) 'Control, confront or collude: How family and society respond to excessive drinking', *British Journal of Addiction*, 87, 1513–25.

Orford, J. and Velleman, R. (1990) 'Offspring of parents with drinking problems: Drinking and drug-taking as young adults', *British Journal of Addiction*, 85, 779–94.

Orford, J., Natera, G., Davies, J., Nava, A., Mora, J., Rigby, K., Bradbury, C., Copello, A. and Velleman, R. (1998) 'Tolerate, engage or withdraw: A study of the structure of families coping with alcohol and drug problems in south-west England and Mexico City', *Addiction*, 93, 1799–813.

Thayer, R. E. (1989) *The biopsychology of mood and arousal*, New York: Oxford University Press.

Wilson, G. W. and Kerr, J. H. (1999) 'Affective responses to success and failure: A study of winning and losing in rugby', *Personality and Individual Differences*, 27, 85–99.

3 Feel the buzz

The positive psychological pay-off from exercise

The late Arthur Lydiard, a New Zealander, was a coach of highly successful distance runners in the 1960s and 1970s. For example, he coached New Zealand athletes Peter Snell and Murray Halberg to victory in the 800-metre and 5,000-metre races in the 1960 Rome Olympics. In 1961, Snell broke three world records in 800-metre, 880-yard and mile races. Ron Clarke, the Australian runner who broke 19 world records in the 1960s, and the very successful group of New Zealand distance runners in the 1970s (Dick Tayler, Rod Dixon, Dick Quax), as well as 1976 Olympic 1,500-metre champion John Walker, all used his basic training methods. During a stay in Finland in 1966–67, Lydiard was also able to influence Finnish coaches and athletes, with Pekka Vasala (1972, 1,500 metres) and Lasse Virén (1972, 1976, 10,000 metres) later producing Olympic gold-winning performances based on his methods. He influenced countless coaches over the years and his training methods are still recognized and used throughout the world of distance running today (Downes, 2004).

Lydiard's training methods involved developing stamina by large amounts of running, strengthening leg muscles by doing hill running and also developing maximum anaerobic capacity by engaging in interval-type training. He was probably the first coach to emphasize the importance of developing high oxygen uptake levels and the importance of tapering down training prior to a race, so that runners are at their peak on their race day. However, in addition to physiological aspects of training, Lydiard was aware of the psychological benefits that can result from running and improved fitness. Long before the popular running boom of the 1970s and 1980s, and the arrival of books such as *The complete book of running* by James Fixx (1977), Lydiard was also using his ideas to improve the fitness, health and well-being of cardiac patients and others in informal 'jogging clubs' (Downes, 2004). He was the real inventor of the concept of jogging, and his greatest legacy is the millions of people around the world who continue to enjoy jogging and running.

It is clear from anecdotal and research evidence that, when people become regular exercisers, taking part in physical activity can have psychological benefits, enhancing their mood and hedonic tone and making them feel better. As Thayer pointed out:

one can hardly speak to a person involved in regular exercise without hearing accounts of beneficial mood changes believed to derive from that exercise. Serious scientists may tend to dismiss these accounts because they are not based on controlled studies, but the consistency of the reports of positive benefits at least suggests that exercise has a powerful influence on mood. In any event, reports by lay people and enthusiasts that mood is strongly affected by exercise are entirely consistent with my research findings.

(Thayer, 1989, p. 93)

This chapter will examine research into the beneficial psychological effects of exercise, or what some (e.g. Biddle and Mutrie, 2001; Kerr, 1997) have called the *feel good factor* associated with exercise. It will outline selected research findings from the general exercise psychology literature (e.g. Biddle and Mutrie, 2001; Ekkekakis and Pettruzello, 1999; Thayer, 1989, 1996) as well as specific findings from reversal theory-based exercise research. The aim will be to show how exercise might play a part in the maintenance and enhancement of arousal, mood and emotion, and go on to show how the psychological benefits obtained from exercise can lead to some exercisers becoming dependent on the exercise-related feel good factor, to the extent that their exercising becomes excessive. As the symptoms of excessive exercising resemble those of other pathological addictions, reference will also be made to Brown's (1997) Hedonic Management Model of Addictions, described in Chapter 2. In addition, reversal theory concepts will be applied to provide an explanation of primary exercise dependence (i.e. exercise dependence without an accompanying eating disorder).

As an aside, it should be stated here that exercise is not for everyone, and some people experience negative or unpleasant psychological consequences from taking part. Often, these unpleasant experiences are associated with initial attempts to exercise, when negative affect or stress may be experienced. It has also been found that some people have experienced social physique anxiety when they have compared their bodily appearance with other exercisers, and increased levels of anxiety have been experienced in those diagnosed with anxiety disorders when exercise intensity has been increased. If the unpleasant experience during the adoption phase becomes too aversive, it is likely to result in the individual abandoning the exercise activity (see e.g. Szabo, 2000).

Exercise research

There have been a few exceptions (e.g. aerobic dance, cycling, swimming, weight training; see e.g. Berger and Motl, 2000), but the vast majority of research studies that have examined the positive effects of exercise have involved running or jogging. This is likely to have been the result of mere expediency on the part of exercise researchers, as there are numerous people involved in running and jogging for exercise and, unlike the majority of other sports, usually no special facilities (e.g. swimming pools, dance studios) or equipment (e.g. weight training equipment, cycling equipment) are required. Nevertheless, a large number of investigations have been undertaken, and Clough *et al.* (1996), for example, counted well over 1,000 articles published in scientific journals on the topic up to that year. In spite of argument and debate and some unresolved difficulties, research evidence in general suggests, and most researchers are convinced, 'that exercise and physical activity participation is consistently associated with positive mood and affect' (Biddle and Mutrie, 2001, p. 201).

Some of the debate has focused on the inadequacy of the methodologies used in a number of early studies and therefore the validity of results obtained. Although many of these early studies were questionable, there were some that were quite adequately designed with sound methodologies and, especially over the last 15 years, there have been numerous additions to this latter group (Berger and Motl, 2000; Biddle and Mutrie, 2001; Ekkekakis and Pettruzello, 1999). For example, Biddle and Mutrie (2001), in their extensive review of physical activity and various aspects of psychological well-being (mood and affect, self-esteem, enjoyment, anxiety, non-clinical depression, cognitive functioning, personality and sleep), stated:

> Much of the debate stems from weak research designs and low statistical power in many studies, thus creating doubt about the true effects of exercise on PWB [psychological well-being]. However, nearly all areas studied show positive effects for exercise across diverse methods of investigation, including meta-analyses, population surveys and experimental trials, and virtually none show negative effects.
>
> (Biddle and Mutrie, 2001, p. 200)

Also central to the debate have been concerns about the exact nature of how exercise works in the process of improved hedonic tone, mood modulation, emotion change and improved psychological well-being. This has led to questions about the effect of various factors, such as the intensity, duration and type of exercise; the fitness and exercise participation levels of study participants (e.g. recreational or competitive); and the choice of laboratory or natural exercise research settings (e.g. Kerr and Kuk, 2001; Kerr *et al.*, 2006). In addition, many of the important issues related to the measures used to assess possible psychological changes in exercisers being tested were discussed in a recent series of papers (Ekkekakis and Petruzzello, 2000, 2001a, 2001b, 2002, 2004; Gauvin and Rejeski, 2001).

Changes in arousal with exercise

As part of the justification for his Hedonic Management Model of Addictions, Brown (1997) claimed that people learn how to manipulate their arousal levels and hedonic tone by engaging in activities that they know will help to decrease the size of any hedonic gap. He included exercise as one of the activities that might be used in this way. Thayer and his colleagues, in several studies, obtained results that showed that even short bouts of exercise (e.g. ten minutes' walking) could increase arousal levels (e.g. Hsiao and Thayer, 1998; Thayer, 1987; Thayer et al., 1987). In addition, there is also evidence available from Thayer's work that people are very adept at using strategies (including exercise) for manipulating arousal levels and moods or emotions in everyday life:

> People use various strategies to modulate their mood from one day to the next, if not from moment to moment. In a number of ways, people attempt to perpetuate their good moods and even to enhance them. And perhaps to an even greater degree, various strategies are regularly employed to eliminate bad moods.
>
> (Thayer 1996, p. 157)

Thayer (1989) put forward a two-dimensional model of mood that was thought to be closely associated with general bodily arousal and that included conscious components of energy (versus tiredness) and tension (versus calmness). These energetic and tense arousal dimensions are to some extent related to the concepts of arousal utilized by Brown (1997) and Apter (1982). In Thayer's theory, energetic arousal and tense arousal can be modulated to optimal levels by individuals self-regulating their own moods. Optimal moods can be realized by means of a self-regulated shift primarily in either arousal dimension or in both dimensions in a complex interaction. Thayer found that individuals use certain strategies and mood regulators (e.g. nicotine, alcohol, sugar or exercise) to manipulate their mood and 'activate' or 'de-activate' themselves (Thayer et al., 1994). This has been termed *personal planning to optimize mood* (Thayer, 1989), or *the self-regulation of mood* (Morris and Reilly, 1987).

Thayer et al. (1994) examined in some detail the strategies that people use to regulate their moods (especially bad or negative moods). They carried out four separate studies that were designed to identify, categorize and evaluate the effectiveness of behaviours commonly used by people to self-regulate their mood. Among their results, they found 32 categories of mood regulation that were used universally by participants to change a bad mood, decrease tension or raise energy. The most frequently used methods to change a bad mood or reduce tension included forms of social interaction and various cognitive techniques. Relaxation and stress management techniques were also found to be used for tense arousal reduction. Rest, splashing water on one's face, getting fresh air and drinking caffeine were found to be commonly used for increasing energetic arousal. However, important in the context of the subject matter of the present book was Thayer et al.'s conclusion about exercise as a strategy for regulating mood:

Of all the separate behavioral categories described to self-regulate mood, a case can be made that exercise is the most effective. This behavior was self-rated as the most successful at changing a bad mood, fourth most successful at raising energy and third or fourth most successful at tension reduction.

(Thayer *et al.*, 1994, p. 921)

A reversal theory-based research investigation involving running (Kerr and Vlaswinkel, 1993) also found that exercise provided the opportunity for arousal modulation. The investigation comprised two field studies that measured changes in arousal in different groups of regularly exercising male and female university students. The exercisers completed the Stress-Arousal Checklist (SACL; Mackay *et al.*, 1978) and the Telic State Measure (TSM; Svebak and Murgatroyd, 1985) before and after running. Male exercisers ran 6.6 kilometres and females 5.0 kilometres on their university campus running trails. Completion times were recorded to allow *fast* and *slow* runners to be compared in the subsequent data analysis (see Table 3.1).

The pre- to post-running results of both field studies showed that male and female groups reported significantly increased scores on experienced or felt arousal. Increases in preferred arousal scores were also obtained for both groups, but these increases only reached significant levels in study 1. Also in study 1, both groups' arousal discrepancy scores (preferred arousal score minus felt arousal score) decreased significantly. These results point to running as being an activity through which exercisers' felt arousal could be increased to desired levels and any discrepancy in arousal levels could be decreased.

In addition, when running times were taken into consideration, fast male (studies 1 and 2) and female fast runners (study 1) reported significantly higher felt arousal scores than slow runners. However, fast males and females in study 2 also had significantly higher preferred arousal scores, and significantly lower arousal discrepancy scores than slow runners, suggesting that these fast runners were more successful than slow runners at attaining their desired levels of arousal and narrowing any experienced discrepancy in arousal levels.

A second reversal theory-based investigation (Kerr and van den Wollenberg, 1997) again involved two field experiments. Different groups of male and female students completed the same short psychological measures pre- and post-exercise as in the Kerr and Vlaswinkel (1993) research. In both experiments, exercisers ran 5.0 kilometres (experiment 1) or 1.7 kilometres (experiment 2) at high (as fast as possible) and low intensities (comfortable, easy speed) on two different occasions as part of a crossover research design (see Table 3.1).

When exercisers' responses to running 5 kilometres and 1.7 kilometres under high and low intensity conditions were compared, arousal scores for male and female groups increased to significantly higher levels when running as fast as possible. When fast and slow runners were compared, fast runners generally achieved higher levels of felt arousal than slow runners. The

Table 3.1 An overview of the research designs used in the reversal theory exercise
field studies and experiments

	Pre-exercise testing	Exercise tasks	Post-exercise testing	Analysis of results
Field Studies 1 of 2 Kerr & Vlaswinkel (1993) (regularly exercising males and females)	TSM and SACL	Males ran 6.6 km Females ran 5 km	TSM and SACL (times recorded)	Comparison of pre- to post-exercise changes; fast vs slow runners
Field Experiment Kerr & vanden Wollenberg (1997) (regularly exercising males and females)	TSM and SACL	Different groups ran 5 km and 1.7 km at high and low intensity – crossover design	TSM and SACL (times recorded)	Comparison of high vs low intensity running; fast vs slow runners
Field Experiment Kerr & Kuk (2001) (regularly exercising males and females)	TESI	Different groups ran 5 km and 1.7 km at high and low intensity – crossover design	TESI (times recorded)	Comparison of pre- to post-exercise changes; high vs low intensity running; fast vs slow runners

results of Kerr and van den Wollenberg's (1997) experiments confirmed the
positive changes in arousal that occurred with exercise found in the other
research described above (Kerr and Vlaswinkel, 1993; Thayer *et al.*, 1994),
but also demonstrated that factors such as distance, running intensity and
personal running ability play a role in the changes that occur in arousal
levels with running.

To summarize, in this section research evidence has been presented which
provides support for the arguments put forward in Brown's (1997) model of
addiction. The fact that exercise has been shown to be an effective way of
allowing individuals to optimize or self-regulate their mood by increasing
arousal levels and/or decreasing any discrepancy between preferred and felt
arousal levels has been demonstrated. This evidence is especially relevant
to the first four stages in the early development of addictions identified by
Brown (1997) and described in Chapter 2.

Changes in emotion with exercise

Much of the discussion in the previous section has been about exercise and
increases in arousal, but the quote from Thayer *et al.* (1994, p. 921) also

underlines the fact that exercise can also serve to reduce tension. A feeling of calm after exercise, resulting from decreases in unpleasant high levels of arousal experienced as anxiety, is what attracts some exercisers. Leith (1994) reviewed some 20 experimental studies and found that 70 per cent showed reductions in anxiety with exercise. Biddle and Mutrie (2001) reviewed a wider range of anxiety studies, including some that used meta-analysis. Based on the findings from these studies, significant small to moderate reductions in anxiety (state, trait and psychophysiological indices of anxiety) were associated with acute and chronic exercise regardless of gender or age. In addition, experimental studies have shown that moderate exercise produces an anxiety-reducing effect, and epidemiological surveys using large populations have supported this anxiety-reducing role (Biddle and Mutrie, 2001).

Among the research studies examining changes in a wider range of emotions with exercise was Kerr and Kuk's (2001) reversal theory investigation using the Tension and Effort Stress Inventory (TESI; e.g. Svebak *et al.*, 1991). Apart from the use of this measure, the research method was identical to that used in the Kerr and van den Wollenberg (1997) research with male and female exercisers running at high and low intensities over distances of 5 kilometres and 1.7 kilometres (see Table 3.1). Although no significant changes in individual emotions were found, groups of pleasant somatic emotions and pleasant transactional emotions were found to increase significantly, while the group of unpleasant somatic emotions (including anxiety) decreased significantly pre- to post-running.

When comparing fast and slow runners in the 5-kilometre run, fast runners reported significantly higher levels of overall pleasant emotions and pleasant transactional emotions than slow runners. Also, for slow runners, running 1.7 kilometres brought about a decrease in total pleasant emotions from pre- to post-running, suggesting that running this distance may have lowered hedonic tone for these runners.

Changes in somatic emotions were expected, as these emotions are based on perceptions of arousal, but the results for transactional emotions were somewhat unexpected. The increases found in pleasant transactional emotions showed that it was possible for exercise to positively affect emotions that concern felt transactional outcome, either self- or other-related, and thus contribute to the improved hedonic tone that exercisers have been found to experience following exercise.

To summarize, it would appear that one of the benefits of exercise is that it can produce changes in emotions, both in terms of broad groups of pleasant or unpleasant emotions and in terms of particular unpleasant emotions such as anxiety. These changes in positive and negative affect can contribute to the 'feel good factor' associated with exercise participation. Part of this may be due to a feeling of calm in the post-exercise recovery phase and beyond, as levels of anxiety and other unpleasant emotions have been reduced by the exercise.

Changes in metamotivational state with exercise

It has been argued above that felt arousal levels and emotions can be modulated by exercise. However, in reversal theory, the experience of emotions is dependent on both the combinations of metamotivational states and the levels of motivational variables (e.g. felt arousal or felt transactional outcome) that are operative at any particular time. Therefore, it should be possible to show that exercise can affect metamotivational states in a manner similar to the changes in state associated with gambling described by Brown (1988).

Objective indices can be used to measure changes in metamotivational state (see e.g. Apter, 1999). For example, Walters *et al.* (1982) established that choosing colours at the blue end of the spectrum was indicative of a preference for low arousal (and therefore the telic state) and choosing colours at the red end was indicative of a preference for high arousal (and therefore the paratelic state). In Kerr and Vlaswinkel's (1993) second field study, described above, in addition to completing psychological measures pre- and post-running, exercisers were asked to make colour choices as they ran. As representative of their arousal preference (rather than actual experienced or felt arousal), runners simply had to indicate either a red or a blue board at the moment they passed a pair of coloured boards prominently displayed at two fixed points on the running trail.

The patterns of preferred arousal obtained in the early stages of the run were slightly different between males and females, but the majority of male and female runners indicated that they were in the telic state. By the end of the run, however, both groups increasingly indicated that they were in the paratelic state and had therefore reversed from the telic to the paratelic state as the run went on. The pattern for fast male runners was similar, but fast females stayed in the telic state for longer than the fast males, even though the majority also found themselves in the paratelic state towards the end of the run. In contrast, while the slow male runners showed a more even balance between telic and paratelic states over the period of the run, the majority of slow female runners started in the paratelic state and remained in that state until the end. Even though some runners remained in the telic state throughout, it is interesting that many of the exercisers were in, or reversed to, the paratelic state, with a preference for high felt arousal, during the run.

Weinberg (1998), using the State of Mind Indicator for Athletes (SOMIFA; Kerr and Apter, 1999), a short psychological measure, studied the predominant metamotivational states and possible reversals in ultra-distance runners in a 100-mile endurance race. Among the items on the SOMIFA are eight statements that correspond to the type of motivation associated with each of the eight metamotivational states (e.g. telic – 'I wanted to achieve something important to me'; paratelic – I wanted simply to enjoy the fun of participating in the event'). Respondents then indicated which one of each pair best described their motivation, reflecting back over the first and second halves of the run. Keeping in mind that the study was restricted to just two measurement points and 156 participants, 1 per cent reversed from the telic to the paratelic state and 25 per cent the opposite way; 6 per cent reversed from the negativistic to the conformist state and 8 per cent the opposite way; 10 per cent reversed from an alloic-mastery state combination to an alloic sympathy state combination and 3 per cent the opposite way; and 1 per cent reversed from an autic-mastery state combination to an autic-sympathy state combination and 12 per cent the opposite way. This study went beyond the Kerr and Vlaswinkel (1993) field study, which was limited to monitoring changes in the telic and paratelic states, to include all the metamotivational states in reversal theory (see Figures A.2 and A.8 in Appendix A). Although some states were more prominent than others, Weinberg (1998) was able to identify that reversals did take place between all the pairs of states.

The results from the two running studies outlined above (Kerr and Vlaswinkel, 1993; Weinberg, 1998), and the findings from several other sport studies (e.g. Bellew and Thatcher, 2002; Fujiyama *et al.*, 2005; Hudson and Bates, 2000; Hudson and Walker, 2002) provide additional support for the notion that psychological reversals do take place in exercise and sport in a fashion similar to those in gambling activities (Brown, 1988, 1997). Therefore, exercise can bring about changes not only in arousal levels and emotions, but also in metamotivational state. To reversal theorists this is not surprising because, according to the theory, the different experience of arousal and emotions is tied in with particular metamotivational states. These concepts have been dealt with separately in the discussion in this chapter merely for convenience. It is important to realize that regular exercisers may actively seek out exercise contexts or situations that allow changes in their operative metamotivational states to take place in planned attempts to modulate arousal levels, trigger certain emotions and generally self-regulate their hedonic tone to optimize pleasant feelings (Kerr, 1997; Thayer, 1996).

Individual experience in exercise activities

While quantitative group-based studies have provided important results that have confirmed the psychological benefits that can accrue from exercise, these studies may have tended to divert attention from the importance of the individual exerciser's unique experience. In this respect, reversal theory would predict that exercise motivation and experience: (a) is likely to vary from person to person; (b) could vary for the same person in exercise sessions over a period of time; and (c) could also vary for an individual exerciser within a particular exercise session. Accounts and descriptions of the personal experience of regular runners can add some credence to these theoretical predictions.

Frey (1993), analysing distance running in reversal theory terms, expanded on the notion that motivation will vary from person to person by providing a list of examples of motives for running that correspond with the theory's various metamotivational categories:

> Runners have different motives for running. They run for fitness (to lose weight, tone muscles, lower blood pressure), to prepare for an upcoming race (a local all-comers track meet or the Boston marathon), to achieve a personal running goal (a 35-minute 10K or a first place in an age division), to escape the pressures and responsibilities of life (a jaunt away from work at lunch hour or away from the kids at home on the weekend), to relish the beauty of nature (a nearby park on a spring morning or an old logging trail on an autumn afternoon), to promote a positive lifestyle change (quit a drug habit), to make decisions and solve problems, to stimulate creative thinking, to cope with depression or anxiety, to acquire a sense of self-mastery or invincibility, to experience passion and intensity, to engage in fantasy, to show off one's body, or to meet a friend or lover.
>
> (Frey, 1993, pp. 157–8)

The type of individual motives listed by Frey (1993) could easily become combined (Kerr, 1997). The example Kerr (1997) used concerned a person who may run to achieve feelings of self-mastery and discipline (autic-mastery), and who does so at a favourite time on a running trail through the woods on a spring morning, enjoying the beauty of nature (paratelic-conformity). In this example the motives for running would be based on a constellation of metamotivational states comprised of paratelic-conformist-autic-mastery.

In addition, motives for exercise could vary for the same person over a period of time. For example, Shyne (1987) described his changing motives for running over a long period and pointed out that:

> I've been running for more than 20 years now, and I know the sport has meant different things to me at different stages of my life. I've run for fitness and health, for friendship and dating, for achievement and self-esteem, for stress control and inspiration . . .
>
> (Shyne, 1987, p. 96)

Reversal theorists would recognize the changing focus of Shyne's (1987) different motives at different stages of his exercise 'career' as representative of the prominence of different states within particular metamotivational state combinations. For example, in running for friendship and dating, the alloic and sympathy states may well have been salient in a combination also involving the paratelic and conformist states, while the salient states when running for achievement and self-esteem would probably have been the autic and mastery states in a state combination of telic-conformist-autic-mastery.

Motives for exercise can also vary for an individual exerciser within a particular exercise session. Frey (1999) gave a retrospective analysis of his own metamotivational experience before, during, and after a 5-mile running road race. Frey's (1999) personal account is an elegant description of the dynamic changes in metamotivation that may take place in exercise situations:

> as the 1500 or so runners began to congregate at the starting line, I reversed momentarily into the *paratelic* state, delighting in the animated horde of runners and jocose announcements made by a city official . . .
>
> The sound of the starter's gun immediately reversed me back into the *telic* state: I started my stopwatch and concentrated on setting a steady pace. Someone in the stampede of runners stepped on my heel, almost pulling my shoe off, prompting me to mutter a *negativistic* comment. His snide retort (something about me slowing faster runners down) left me in this state for most of the first mile.
>
> I ran most of the remainder of the race in a *telic/mastery* frame of mind. Once the field of runners thinned out, I encountered a series of one-on-one 'battles' – which always found me in the *autic* and *mastery* states . . . Several times a runner near me dropped off to the side, apparently quitting the race. While I clearly felt *mastery*-oriented pride in passing one such runner, I reversed briefly into the *alloic* state in response to another such runner.
>
> The first three miles were all clearly marked – allowing me to *telicly* monitor my progress during the race. However, I did not see (or perhaps missed) the fourth mile marker. The gradual realization of this as the fourth mile seemed to drag endlessly on reversed me to the *negativistic* state ('incompetent race organizers,' I thought).
>
> Although I remained *telic* throughout most of the final mile, I experienced an obvious reversal to the *paratelic* state as I neared the finish line and felt buoyed by the boisterous crowd (which had cheered the first-place finisher nearly five minutes earlier).
>
> (Frey, 1999, p. 15)[1]

These personal accounts illustrate the dynamic nature of motivation for exercise, including the salience of the various operative states, and ongoing reversals between pairs of states during exercise, but can this metamotivational diversity contribute to a person's psychological well-being?

As it happens, relatively frequent reversals, having all eight states operative and experiencing the full palette of emotions over time is considered to be a mark of psychological health and well-being in reversal theory (Apter, 1989/2006; Lafreniere *et al.*, 2001). It does not require a huge leap of faith to realize that, 'if exercise works for them', some individuals could deliberately begin to use exercise as a means of boosting their psychological health and well-being in their daily lives. Once a person discovers the potential of exercise to make them feel better, then it is just a small step for those whose exercise adherence level is high to begin using exercise deliberately as an effective means of modulating arousal and/or prompting reversals to maintain improved well-being. Most individuals may be content to engage in exercise activities for this purpose in relative moderation, but some may find themselves taking their need for enhanced hedonic tone a few stages further and developing a fully fledged behavioural addiction. Kerr (1997) stated:

> While there is a positive side to participation in sports and exercise activities, in terms of satisfying the needs of particular states (or state combinations) and contributing to the maintenance of an individual's metamotivational and emotional equilibrium, there is another side to the coin. Some individuals may use exercise to replace and improve upon other types of arousal and mood modulation strategies. These individuals appear to have discovered that continuous use of excessive levels of exercise and sport activities can provide a relatively reliable and effective means of manipulating hedonic tone in the directions they desire (see Brown, 1997). However, these individuals run the risk of becoming dependent on, or addicted to, sports and exercise activities in what Glasser (1976) has called a *positive addiction*.
>
> (Kerr, 1997, p. 141)

Glasser's (1976) term 'positive addiction' is actually a misnomer. He used this term because regular exercise is generally associated with good health and therefore considered positive in comparison with other more destructive addictions that have severe negative consequences. However, like other addictions, exercise addiction can also have negative consequences for the health and well-being of the individual (e.g. Szabo, 2000).

The final section of the chapter reviews some of the reversal theory interpretations of primary exercise addiction (Kerr, 1997). Readers unfamiliar with reversal theory are again directed to Appendix A for clarification of reversal theory terms and concepts.

Primary exercise dependence through the lens of reversal theory

Kerr (1997) speculated on the likely metamotivational style of those people who are exercise dependent. He pointed out that endurance type activities, often associated with exercise dependence (e.g. running, cycling, swimming, aerobics and weight training; see Chapter 1), are especially attractive to telic dominant individuals (those who are frequently in the telic state), for at least two reasons. First, these types of activities satisfy their desire to achieve essential and (for them) unavoidable goals by, for example, attaining certain times, distances, weights or repetitions. Second, endurance exercise often involves a large time commitment and has to be carefully planned within a person's other daily and weekly tasks and commitments. Both the need for planning and the successful outcome of that planning appeal to the telic dominant person, and provide pleasant feelings of satisfaction and improved hedonic tone.

Research results have shown that those who take part in relatively safe endurance sports were significantly more telic dominant than participants in explosive or risk sports (Kerr and Svebak, 1989; Svebak and Kerr, 1989). Of course, very few telic dominant sports performers will necessarily become exercise dependent, but there is a danger that exercise activities may become merely an extension of their telic-dominant lifestyle, to the point where they may take over (Apter, 1990).

With regard to the other metamotivational pairs, the pattern of conformist, autic and mastery dominance proposed by Kerr (1997) is also likely to feature strongly in the addicted exerciser's motivational style. In addition, exercise activities have many aspects or characteristics which are attractive to individuals with this type of motivational style. For example, with the need to comply with planned exercise schedules and complete hours of exercise activities on a very regular basis, conformity, rather than negativism dominance, is likely. On occasion, the need to conform to exercise requirements may even become a threat to the exerciser's health and well-being, where they may attempt to follow their punishing exercise regimes when ill or injured. This was true of Jiu-Jitsu athlete Joanna (Griffiths, 1997) described in Chapter 2. Joanna also exhibited a tendency to focus on herself at the expense of others, including her partner and friends. This indicates that addicted exercisers are likely to become increasingly autic dominant and have the self-oriented autic state operative for much of the time, rather than the other-oriented alloic state. The mastery state is thought to make up the fourth part of an addicted exerciser's likely motivational style profile (Kerr, 1997). Research findings have shown that exercise activities may provide the opportunity for addicted exercisers to exert a degree of control over their own bodies and their life in general, improving their self-esteem, feelings of competence and even self-identity (e.g. Robbins and Joseph, 1985; Yates, 1991; Yates et al., 1983). Kerr (1997) concluded that the addicted exerciser's motivational style profile was likely to be characterized by telic, conformist, autic and mastery dominance. These arguments were tested in a series of studies (Blaydon, 2001; Blaydon and Lindner, 2002; Blaydon et al., 2002, 2004). The results of these studies will be reviewed in Chapters 6 and 7.

Kerr (1997) also argued that, in trying to understand how and why exercise dependence can occur, there are three likely reversal theory explanations of the motivational processes involved. The first involves the management of hedonic tone through arousal modulation outlined by Brown (1997, 2001), and the second and third involve reversal problems associated with reversal inhibition described by Murgatroyd and Apter (1984, 1986) and by Miller (1985).

Anxiety reduction

Given that addicted exercisers are likely to be in the telic and conformity states for longer periods than their paired partner states, it is possible that exercise is used to reduce unpleasantly high levels of felt arousal to lower levels where it can be experienced as relaxation. Research has shown that anxiety levels are often reduced after exercise (see e.g. Ekkekakis and Petruzello, 1999; McAuley *et al.*, 1996; Morgan, 1987). However, because the autic and mastery states are also likely to be operative, overall hedonic tone may receive a further boost from feelings of pride arising from increased felt transactional outcome as the exerciser realizes that, for example, he or she has completed the swim in a faster time or cycled further than before. In other words, exercise is used as a strategy to improve hedonic tone by arousal reduction and by enhancing felt transactional outcome. Over time, this hedonic management strategy may become less effective as addicted exercisers become tolerant to the exercise activity, and they may have to exercise with greater intensity and for longer periods to produce the same improved levels of hedonic tone after exercise.

Reversal inhibition: achieving satisfaction

Addicted exercisers may experience problems reversing in everyday life because of what Miller (1985) called *rigidity or imbalance* and Apter (e.g. 1989) *reversal inhibition*. This means that they are 'stuck' or 'trapped' in a particular combination of states most of the time, with only very occasional reversals to other state(s). Experiencing the full range of metamotivational states over time is thought to be necessary for maintaining psychological health (Apter, 1989/2006). If reversals do not occur relatively frequently between partner states, it may cause psychological disturbance and problems may arise (e.g. Kerr *et al.*, 1993; Lafreniere *et al.*, 2001).

Excessive levels of exercise may thus become necessary to maintain emotional equilibrium in the individual who is experiencing reversal inhibition. For example, for the individual who spends most of the time trapped in the telic-conformist-autic-mastery state combination, sport and exercise may be a, or perhaps the only, means for that individual to achieve pleasure and satisfaction in life (Apter, 1989, p. 145). For this type of addicted exerciser, the completion of previously planned schedules and exercise regimes, along with personal goal achievement as exercise targets are set, reached and reset, and the feelings of personal control from domination of mind over body, can provide tremendous satisfaction and enhanced hedonic tone.

Reversal inhibition: facilitating reversals

Another possibility is that excessive exercise helps to facilitate reversals in those who are experiencing reversal inhibition, and exercise addicts become reliant on the addictive behaviour to bring about reversals (Brown, 2001; Miller, 1985). Take, for example, an individual trapped in the telic-conformist-autic-mastery state combination with the telic state salient, experiencing high felt arousal and suffering from chronic anxiety, one of the psychological problems arising from inhibited reversals (Apter, 1982; Lafreniere *et al.*, 2001). Excessive exercise may have become the only possible means for these individuals to trigger a reversal. In this case, a reversal from the telic to the paratelic state might allow them some respite from their chronic anxiety as the high arousal is reinterpreted as pleasant excitement (Apter, 1989, p. 151). This change may occur during exercise and perhaps endure for some time afterwards, before a reversal back to the telic state. Inducing reversals in this way as a strategy for improving hedonic tone may become more and more difficult, and the individuals concerned may also have to take part in increasingly more intense and more frequent exercise activities to provoke reversals in the future.

These three possible explanations of the motivational processes involved in exercise dependence are speculative (Kerr, 1997) and need to be explored in detail with individuals who are exercise dependent. The qualitative work involving interviews, reviewed in Chapter 7, may help to shed some light on which of the possible explanations are credible.

Closing comments

One of the purposes of this chapter was to show how exercise can have beneficial effects and play a part in the maintenance and enhancement of individual well-being. Early in the chapter, considerable space was given to explaining how exercise could be used to modulate arousal levels, change a person's state of mind and/or bring about changes in emotions, all with the goal of improving hedonic tone. Some selected research findings were presented to support this notion.

A second purpose was to show how the psychological high or 'feel good factor' obtained from exercise can become problematic in some cases, with individuals becoming addicted to, or dependent on, the improvements in hedonic tone provided by exercise. Building on the previous research on addictions in general, explored in Chapter 2, exercise addiction was examined through the lens of reversal theory, and some interesting explanations from Miller (1985) and from Murgatroyd and Apter's (1984, 1986) psychotherapeutic work on reversal problems were applied to exercise addiction.

At this point in the book, it is necessary to leave temporarily the analysis of primary exercise dependence and proceed to investigate eating disorders. Chapter 4 will explain exactly what eating disorders are and how they develop, and probe the link between these disorders and exercise. Chapter 5 will discuss eating disorders in athlete populations and then go on to consider secondary exercise dependence.

Notes

1 Source: 'Reversal theory: Basic concepts' by K. Frey, in J. H. Kerr (ed.) *Experiencing sport: Reversal theory*. Copyright 1999 John Wiley & Sons Limited. Reprinted with permission.

References

Apter, M. J. (1982) *The experience of motivation*, London: Academic Press.

Apter, M. J. (1989) *Reversal theory: Motivation, emotion and personality*, London: Routledge. (2nd edition published 2006.)

Apter, M. J. (1990) 'Sport and mental health: A new psychological perspective', in G. P. H. Hermans and W. L. Mosterd (eds) *Sports, medicine and health*, Amsterdam: Elsevier, 47–56.

Apter, M. J. (1999) 'Measurement challenges in reversal theory sport research', in J. H. Kerr (ed.) *Experiencing sport: Reversal theory*, Chichester: Wiley, 19–36.

Apter, M. J. (2006) *Reversal theory: The dynamics of motivation, emotion and personality*, 2nd edition, Oxford: Oneworld Publications.

Bellew, E. and Thatcher, J. (2002) 'Metamotivational state reversals in competitive sport', *Social Behavior and Personality*, 30, 613–24.

Berger, B. G. and Motl, R. W. (2000) 'Exercise and mood: A selective review and synthesis of research employing the Profile of Mood States', *Journal of Applied Sport Psychology*, 12, 69–92.

Biddle, S. J. H. and Mutrie, N. (2001) *Psychology of physical activity*, London: Routledge.

Blaydon, M. J. (2001) 'Descriptive and metamotivational characteristics of primary and secondary exercise dependent and eating disordered participants in intense physical activity', unpublished PhD thesis, Hong Kong: University of Hong Kong.

Blaydon, M. J. and Lindner, K. J. (2002) 'Eating disorders and exercise dependence in triathletes', *Eating Disorders*, 10, 49–60.

Blaydon, M. J., Lindner, K. J. and Kerr, J. H. (2002) 'Metamotivational characteristics of eating-disordered and exercise-dependent triathletes', *Psychology of Sport and Exercise*, 3, 223–36.

Blaydon, M. J., Lindner, K. J. and Kerr, J. H. (2004) 'Metamotivational characteristics of exercise dependence and eating disorders in highly active amateur sport participants', *Personality and Individual Differences*, 36, 1419–32.

Brown, R. I. F. (1988) 'Reversal theory and subjective experience in the explanation of addiction and relapse', in M. J. Apter, J. H. Kerr and M. P. Cowles (eds) *Progress in reversal theory*, Amsterdam: Elsevier, 191–212.

Brown, R. I. F. (1997) 'A theoretical model of behavioural addictions – Applied to offending', in J. E. Hodge, M. McMurran and C. R. Hollin (eds) *Addicted to crime?*, New York: Wiley, 13–65.

Brown, R. I. F. (2001) 'Addictions', in M. J. Apter (ed.) *Motivational styles in everyday life: A guide to reversal theory*, Washington DC: American Psychological Association, 155–65.

Clough, P., Hockey, B. and Sewell, D. (1996) 'The use of a diary methodology to assess the impact of exercise on mental states', in C. Robson, B. Cripps and H. Steinberg (eds) *Quality and quantity: Research methods in sport and exercise psychology*, Leicester: British Psychological Society, 22–7.

Downes, S. (2004) 'Arthur Lydiard', *The Independent*, 15 December. Online. Available http//:news.independent.co.uk.

Ekkekakis, P. and Petruzzello, S. J. (1999) 'Acute aerobic exercise and affect: Current status, problems and prospects regarding dose-response', *Sports Medicine*, 28, 337–74.

Ekkekakis, P. and Petruzzello, S. J. (2000) 'Analysis of the affect measurement conundrum in exercise psychology: I. Fundamental issues', *Psychology of Sport and Exercise*, 1, 71–88.

Ekkekakis, P. and Petruzzello, S. J. (2001a) Analysis of the affect measurement conundrum in exercise psychology: II. A conceptual and methodological critique of the Exercise-induced Feeling Inventory. *Psychology of Sport and Exercise*, 2, 1–26.

Ekkekakis, P. and Petruzzello, S. J. (2001b) 'Analysis of the affect measurement conundrum in exercise psychology: III. A conceptual and methodological critique of the Subjective Exercise Experiences Scale', *Psychology of Sport and Exercise*, 2, 205–32.

Ekkekakis, P. and Petruzzello, S. J. (2002) 'Analysis of the affect measurement conundrum in exercise psychology: IV. A conceptual case for the affect circumplex', *Psychology of Sport and Exercise*, 3, 35–63.

Ekkekakis, P. and Petruzzello, S. J. (2004) 'Affective, but hardly effective: A reply to Gauvin and Rejeski (2001)', *Psychology of Sport and Exercise*, 5, 135–52.

Fixx, J. F. (1977) *The complete book of running*, New York: Random House.

Frey, K. (1993) 'Distance running: A reversal theory analysis', in J. H. Kerr, S. Murgatroyd and M. J. Apter (eds) *Advances in reversal theory*, Amsterdam: Swets and Zeitlinger, 157–64.

Frey, K. (1999) 'Reversal theory: Basic concepts', in J. H. Kerr (ed.) *Experiencing sport: Reversal theory*, Chichester: Wiley, 3–17.

Fujiyama, H., Wilson, G. and Kerr, J. H. (2005) 'Motivational state and emotional tone in baseball: The reciprocity between reversal theory and field research', *European Review of Applied Psychology*, 55, 71–83.

Gauvin, L. and Rejeski, W. J. (2001) 'Disentangling substance from rhetoric: A rebuttal to Ekkekakis and Petruzzello (2001)', *Psychology of Sport and Exercise*, 2, 73–88.

Glasser, W. (1976) *Positive addiction*, New York: Harper and Row.

Griffiths, M. (1997) 'Exercise addiction: A case study', *Addiction Research and Theory*, 5, 161–8.

Hsiao, E. T. and Thayer, R. E. (1998) 'Exercising for mood regulation: The importance of experience', *Personality and Individual Differences*, 24, 829–36.

Hudson, J. and Bates, M. D. (2000) 'Factors affecting metamotivational reversals during motor task performance', *Perceptual and Motor Skills*, 91, 373–84.

Hudson, J. and Walker, N. (2002) 'Metamotivational state reversals during matchplay golf: An idiographic approach', *The Sport Psychologist*, 16, 200–17.

Kerr, J. H. (1997) *Motivation and emotion in sport: Reversal theory*, Hove: Psychology Press.

Kerr, J. H. and Apter, M. J. (1999) 'The State of Mind Indicator for Athletes', in J. H. Kerr (ed.) *Experiencing sport: Reversal theory*, Chichester: Wiley, 239–44.

Kerr, J. H. and Kuk, G. (2001) 'The effects of low and high intensity exercise on emotions, stress and effort', *Psychology of Sport and Exercise*, 2, 173–86.

Kerr, J. H. and Svebak (1989) 'Motivational aspects of preference for and participation in risk sports', *Personality and Individual Differences*, 10, 797–800.

Kerr, J. H. and van den Wollenberg, A. E. (1997) High and low intensity exercise and psychological mood states, *Psychology and Health*, 12, 603–18.

Kerr, J. H. and Vlaswinkel, E. H. (1993) 'Self-reported mood and running', *Work and Stress*, 7, 161–77.

Kerr, J. H., Frank-Regan, E. and Brown, R. I. F. (1993) 'Taking risks with health', *Patient Guidance and Counseling*, 22, 73–80.

Kerr, J. H., Fujiyama, H., Sugano, A., Okamura, T., Chang, M. and Onouha, F. (2006) 'Psychological responses to exercising in laboratory and natural environments', *Psychology of Sport and Exercise*, 7, 345–59.

Lafreniere, K. D., Ledgerwood, D. M. and Murgatroyd, S. J. (2001) 'Psychopathology, therapy and counseling', in M. J. Apter (ed.) *Motivational styles in everyday life: A guide to reversal theory*, Washington: American Psychological Association, 263–85.

Leith, L. (1994) *Foundations of exercise and mental health*, Morgantown VA: Fitness Information Technology.

McAuley, E., Mihalko, S. L. and Bane, S. M. (1996) 'Acute exercise and anxiety reduction: Does the environment matter?', *Journal of Sport and Exercise Psychology*, 18, 408–19.

Mackay, C. J., Cox, T., Burrows, G. C. and Lazzerini, A. J. (1978) 'An inventory for the measurement of self-reported stress and arousal', *British Journal of Social and Clinical Psychology*, 17, 283–4.

Miller, W. R. (1985) 'Addictive behaviour and the theory of psychological reversals', *Addictive Behaviors*, 10, 177–180.

Morgan, W. P. (1987) 'Reduction of state anxiety following acute physical activity', in W. P. Morgan and S. E. Goldston (eds) *Exercise and mental health*, Washington DC: Hemisphere Publishing, 105–9.

Morris, W. N. and Reilly, N. P. (1987) 'Toward the self-regulation of mood: Theory and research', *Motivation and Emotion*, 11, 215–49.

Murgatroyd, S. and Apter, M. J. (1984) 'Eclectic psychotherapy: A structural phenomenological approach', in W. R. Dryden (ed.) *Individual psychotherapy in Britain*, London: Harper and Row, 389–414.

Murgatroyd, S. and Apter, M. J. (1986) 'A structural-phenomenological approach to eclectic psychotherapy', in J. Norcross (ed.) *Casebook of eclectic psychotherapy*, New York: Bruner/Mazel, 260–80.

Robbins, J. M. and Joseph, P. (1985) 'Experiencing exercise withdrawal: Possible consequences of therapeutic and mastery running', *Journal of Sport Psychology*, 7, 23–39.

Shyne, K. (1987) 'Paternal instincts', *Runners World*, 96, December. Cited in Frey, K. (1993) 'Distance running: A reversal theory analysis', in J. H. Kerr, S. Murgatroyd and M. J. Apter (eds) *Advances in reversal theory*, Amsterdam: Swets and Zeitlinger, 158.

Svebak, S. and Murgatroyd, S. (1985) 'Metamotivational dominance: A multi-method validation of reversal theory constructs', *Journal of Personality and Social Psychology*, 48, 107–16.

Svebak, S. and Kerr, J. H. (1989) 'The role of impulsivity in preference for sports', *Personality and Individual Differences*, 10, 1, 51–8.

Svebak, S., Ursin, H., Endresen, I., Hjelmen, A. M. and Apter, M. J. (1991) 'Psychological factors in the aetiology of back pain', *Psychology and Health*, 5, 307–14.

Szabo, A. (2000) 'Physical activity as a source of psychological dysfunction', in S. J. H. Biddle, K. R. Fox and S. H. Boutcher (eds) *Physical activity and psychological well-being*, London: Routledge, 130–95.

Thayer, R. E. (1987) 'Energy, tiredness and tension effects of a sugar snack versus moderate exercise', *Journal of Personality and Social Psychology*, 52, 119–25.

Thayer, R. E. (1989) *The biopsychology of mood and arousal*, New York: Oxford University Press.

Thayer, R. E. (1996) *The origin of everyday moods*, New York: Oxford University Press.

Thayer, R. E., Peters, D. P., Takahashi, P. J. and Birkhead-Flight, A. M. (1987) 'Mood and behavior (smoking and sugar snacking) following moderate exercise: A partial test of Self-Regulation Theory', *Personality and Individual Differences*, 14, 97–104.

Thayer, R. E., Newman, J. R. and McClain, T. M. (1994) 'The self-regulation of mood: Strategies for changing a bad mood, raising energy, and reducing tension', *Journal of Personality and Social Psychology*, 67, 910–25.

Walters, J., Apter, M. J. and Svebak, S. (1982) 'Color preference, arousal and the theory of psychological reversals', *Motivation and Emotion*, 6, 193–215.

Weinberg, G. M. (1998) 'Motivation in ultra distance runners: A reversal theory approach to optimal experience', unpublished PhD thesis, Santa Barbara CA: Fielding Institute.

Yates, A., (1991) *Compulsive exercise and the eating disorders*, New York: Brunner Mazel.

Yates, A., Leehey, K. and Shisslak, C. M. (1983) 'Running: An analogue of anorexia?', *New England Journal of Medicine*, 308, 251–5.

4 Driven to be thin
Eating disorders and how they develop

The fashion industry, with its preoccupation with extremely thin female models, is often accused of presenting the wrong body image to young girls who, in striving to achieve this image, may engage in unhealthy eating habits and put themselves at risk of developing eating disorders (e.g. Brownell, 1991; Davis *et al.*, 2000). It is perhaps ironic, therefore, that a member of a high-profile media fashion family should have recently written about her struggle with an eating disorder (Lauren, 2005). Jenny Lauren, niece of well-known fashion designer Ralph Lauren, admitted to having suffered from the eating disorder bulimia, coupled with excessive exercise.

She began as a child model for the fashion firm and took part in ballet training in her early years. At the age of 14, unhappy with her body image, she began starving herself, and by the age of 15 she was 5 feet 4 inches tall and weighed 84 pounds, a weight similar to that of many of the thinnest dancers and models. Shortly afterwards, she started vomiting and purging and became a fully fledged bulimic. At one point she required hospitalization. Later, while at college, she started exercising to excess and this became inextricably linked with her bulimia:

> I had a routine: running every morning in Central Park, then fitting in callisthenics before I showered and went to class. Then roaming the college cafeteria for something without oil to eat. Then being hungry the rest of the day while I sat through my other classes. Then rushing to a power yoga class, where I felt like I might pass out during a sun salutation. Then home, where I'd have to write a whole paper that I'd put off in order to keep up my exercise schedule. And then the vomiting.
> ... Still, I kept punishing my body, even when I started having agonizing spasms in my bowels. I saw doctor after doctor, and no one could determine what was wrong. After months of embarrassing tests and the best specialists telling me to get a shrink, a surgeon finally discovered the problem. My mom, dad and I sat in his office and stared dumbfounded, at a set of X-rays that showed my small intestines resting in the middle of my rectum and vagina. I asked the surgeon if I had caused my condition. He hesitated and softly said: 'Well you may have

a congenital weakness, but it's more likely the result of straining from your eating disorder'.

(Lauren, 2005, p. 2)

Lauren was told that if she did not have surgery she would probably become incontinent. However, despite two surgeries, she continues to suffer from chronic pain. Having conquered her eating disorder ('I can't even remember the last time I tried to make myself throw up' [Lauren, 2005, p. 2]), she claims to be happier now than in her teenage years and is unconcerned about how she looks. Based on the definitions and explanations provided in Chapter 1, Lauren's case illustrates a progression from an eating disorder to an eating disorder with exercise dependence in her college years. Her exercise dependence appears to have been secondary to her bulimia (De Coverly Veale, 1987; Veale, 1995). This chapter will focus on eating disorders such as Lauren's bulimia, explaining how they develop, providing descriptions and definitions of their main characteristics, the criteria for their diagnosis and descriptive examples.

Eating disorders

The National Collaboration Centre for Mental Health (NCCMH) in the UK is a partnership between the Royal College of Psychiatrists' Research Unit and the British Psychological Society's Centre for Outcomes Research and Effectiveness. In 2004, an NCCMH report containing national guidelines for clinical practice for eating disorders was published (NCCMH, 2004). A reference group of 13 different organizations concerned with eating disorders provided advice on a full range of issues related to the development of the guidelines. The guidelines represent a UK consensus of opinion on core interventions in the treatment and management of anorexia nervosa, bulimia nervosa and related eating disorders, and much of the information below about these eating disorders comes from that document. Other recent sources of information on anorexia nervosa and bulimia nervosa include Cooper (2003) and Lucas (2004).

According to the NCCMH, about 1 in 250 females (0.4 per cent) and 1 in 2,000 males (0. 05 per cent) experience anorexia nervosa; five times that number suffer from bulimia nervosa. Other estimations from epidemiological research suggest that the average prevalence rate in young females for anorexia nervosa is 0.3 per cent and 1 per cent for bulimia nervosa (Van Hoeken *et al.*, 2005). It is estimated that males make up approximately 10 per cent of those who present with anorexia and bulimia, and 25 per cent of those who present with binge eating disorder (American Psychiatric Association (APA), 1994; Fairburn and Beglin, 1990). Among adolescents, anorexia has the highest mortality rate of any psychiatric disorder and depression is a common comorbid diagnosis, with rates of up to 63 per cent in some studies (Herzog *et al.*, 1992).

Anorexia nervosa

According to the NCCMH report (2004), anorexia nervosa often starts with some form of dieting behaviour. In some people it may develop through purging rather than dieting. Over time, restriction of food intake becomes more and more stringent and precisely defined as control over weight is a priority. Individuals with anorexia often perceive themselves to be fatter than they actually are. Consequently, the positive achievement and experience of weight loss provides strong reinforcement to these individuals who are also likely to be experiencing low self-confidence and self-esteem. As the condition becomes more serious, it may be accompanied by social withdrawal, rigidity and obsessionality. In addition, emotional disturbance in the form of increasing anxiety and mood disturbance will become apparent as the condition develops (e.g. Cooper and Bowskill, 1986; NCCMH, 2004).

The physical consequences of anorexia, depending on the intensity and duration of the anorexia, can become so severe that every system in the body is affected. These problems can range from general lethargy, fatigue and lack of energy to cessation of menstruation, loss of sexual desire, and even infertility, and can also include loss of muscle strength, loss of bone density, permanent stunting of growth, and detrimental effects on the endocrine system. Eventually, anorexia will start to have a negative effect on a person's life in general, with detrimental effects on education, work and leisure. In the NCCMH guidelines anorexia nervosa is defined as:

> A syndrome in which the individual maintains a low weight as a result of preoccupation with body weight, construed either as a fear of fatness or pursuit of thinness. Weight is maintained at least 15 per cent below that expected or body mass index (calculated as weight in kilograms divided by height in metres squared) is below 17.5. Weight loss is self-induced by exercise, vomiting or purgation, and avoidance of fattening foods. A widespread endocrine disorder involving the hypothalamo-pituitary-gonadal axis is present. In females this is manifest as amenorrhoea and in males by loss of sexual interest and impotence. Other psychosocial features such as mood disorder, obsessive-compulsive symptoms and social withdrawal are common.
>
> (NCCMH, 2004, p. 254)

An example of the type of behaviour and thinking associated with anorexia was provided by Epstein (1993). The case of Madelyn, who tried to keep to a 150-calorie-a-day diet, illustrates the very precise thinking about amounts of food that is common among anorexics:

> When I was 12 I put myself on a diet. I would drink one glass of powdered skim milk and eat one hard-boiled egg. I would eat an egg because that

was a measured amount, and I used to agonize over the size of the egg after a while ... One night I was dragged to a relative's house for dinner. I remember eating a piece of lettuce and feeling that the whole month and a half was for nothing, that my diet had been ruined. I wanted to kill myself. I felt very out of control.

(Epstein, 1993, p. 60)

Another example of the role of 'control' emphasized by Madelyn was provided by Diane Hague (1987), writing about her own seven-year struggle with eating disorders. Her anorexia lasted two years and then she developed bulimia:

I was 22 at the time. I ate one meal a day. I was very, very disciplined. I restricted myself to 800 calories a day and no more. I would count every single calorie. One calorie over and I'd be very unhappy for the rest of the day. I never ate breakfast and I'd skip lunch. For my evening meal, I'd have something like toast, coffee and bananas, or rather one banana. My weight had dropped from about eight and a half stone to five stone, and I still thought I was very fat ... I was hyperactive. I'd sleep about three hours a night ...

When I was anorexic, I was at least feeling good about myself. I felt as if I was in control of my own body. I was, of course, deceiving everybody around me about the amount I was actually eating. But it was me that was controlling what I was eating. With bulimia I felt totally out of control.

(Hague, 1987, p. 1)

It is interesting that Hague (1987) eventually came to terms with her eating disorders by taking up marathon running as therapy. Running made her 'feel good' and more self-confident, and she learned that, through exercise, she could control her body without using laxatives and forced vomiting. However, she also admitted that she became just as compulsive about exercise as she was about food, running six days and covering 70 miles a week.

Bulimia nervosa

There is evidence of a strong relationship between anorexia and bulimia, with over 25 per cent of patients with bulimia having experienced an episode of anorexia (Shafran and de Silva, 2005). Repeated episodes of binge eating followed by reactive compensatory behaviour designed to prevent putting on weight are the main characteristics of bulimia. These episodes of binge eating are frequently planned, with the individuals buying or preparing large amounts of food for consumption without interruption. Bulimics, however, are generally able to maintain their weight at normal levels by, for example, engaging in compensatory purging to offset the possible weight gains brought about by eating binges. The post-binge compensatory behaviour may take the form of self-induced vomiting, purging, fasting or excessive exercising, either separately or in combination. The misuse of laxatives, diuretics, thyroxine, amphetamine or other types of medication may be involved (NCCMH, 2004). Like anorexics, bulimics tend to be secretive about this behaviour, which generally progresses into a cycle of attempted dieting, binge eating and compensatory behaviour.

Psychologically, bulimics tend to be over-concerned with body shape and weight, and experience low self-esteem and physical self-loathing, much like anorexics. The negative emotions of anxiety and tension are frequently experienced, and mood disturbance is also very common. Bulimics often have the feeling that they have lost control when they engage in binge eating episodes. Although often experiencing an emotional high during a binge, they typically experience unpleasant feelings of shame and guilt afterwards. This unpleasant emotional experience is often exacerbated and reinforced by the comments of family members or others.

Physical problems are generally less serious than those found with anorexics, but often include fatigue, lethargy, feeling bloated, constipation, abdominal pain, swelling of hands and feet, irregular menstruation and the erosion of tooth enamel. In addition to abnormalities in the menstrual cycle, bulimia may affect other aspects of the endocrine system, including the release of thyroid-stimulating hormone and growth hormone response to the thyroid-stimulating hormone (NCCMH, 2004). In severe cases, such as that of Jenny Lauren, irreversible damage to the internal organs may result. In some cases, bulimic episodes may occur daily, and through time bulimia tends to reorganize and dominate daily life. Social and relationship problems may develop. In the NCCMH guidelines, bulimia nervosa was defined as:

> A syndrome characterized by recurrent episodes of binge eating and by compensatory behaviour (vomiting, purging, fasting or exercising) in order to prevent weight gain. Binge eating is accompanied by a subjective feeling of loss of control over eating. This is a normal weight syndrome in which body mass index (BMI) is maintained above 17.5 kg/m² in adults and the equivalent in children and adolescents.
>
> (NCCMH, 2004, p. 254)

By way of illustration, Wijesinghe (1977) described a typical binge-eating episode in a 37-year-old woman with a six-year eating problem:

> At the beginning of an episode she would have sensations which she described as 'feverish excitement' which would compel her to go to the nearest baker's shop and buy large quantities of sweet, starchy foods – cakes, biscuits, chocolates – and either drive out in her car to some secluded place or take the food home. She would then set about consuming this food in a voracious manner 'making a pig of myself' as

she put it. This would continue for an hour or two, by which time she would feel 'bloated, tired and sick'. This would usually be followed by loss of appetite for a day or two, whilst she would feel extremely guilty. The abstinence from food after a compulsive eating episode kept her weight within bounds. Nevertheless it seriously disrupted her work ... and also her social life.

(Wijesinghe, 1977, p. 86)

Table 4.1 shows the contents of a monitoring sheet completed by a patient with bulimia. It provides more comprehensive details of what was consumed, the time scale, subsequent vomiting or laxative use and details the feelings associated with the bulimic's eating binges (Fairburn *et al.*, 1990).

Lam (2001) has reported part of a conversation he had during treatment sessions with a client, which focused on a recent binge-purge situation. Rachel, the client, was an attractive and intelligent woman in her early thirties who worked for an international company, and this entailed frequent travel abroad. She described herself as reasonably successful, but in spite of this she had low self-esteem and was not assertive. She said she was a sensitive person who felt secure only when she felt accepted by almost everyone. She said she was something of a perfectionist and felt very dissatisfied when she could not attain the very high standards she set for herself both in many aspects of her life and in her intense dieting. After a business lunch where she perceived that she had eaten too much, she became anxious and angry with herself for not being able to control the amount of food that she ate; she also felt guilty about her lack of control. After the incident, Rachel cut down her eating, used laxatives and exercised more than usual over the following days. The conversation, part of the 'cognitive assessment process' in a cognitive behaviour therapy approach to helping Rachel with her bulimia, is reproduced in part below (*T* = Therapist; *C* = Client):

T: What was so anxious-provoking in your mind about 'eating too much' in the restaurant?

C: I don't want to.

T: I know you don't want to, but what was going through your mind when you believed that you had too much to eat.

C: I will be fat.

T: Suppose, let me just suppose that you are fat, then what?

C: Ugly.

T: What if you are ugly?

C: I don't like to be ugly.

T: I wonder why?

C: That means I am losing control, and I don't want that to happen.

T: What will it mean to you about losing control?

C: I will not be liked by people, if that is the case.

T: Who are these people?

Table 4.1 A monitoring sheet illustrating the eating habits of a patient with bulimia nervosa (it is typical of a patient in the early states of treatment)

Time	Food and liquid consumed	Place	B	V/P	Circumstances
					Date 7th November Day Wednesday
7.45	1 apple 1 grapefruit 1 black coffee	kitchen			Depressed. Feel fat
3.10	1 egg sandwich 1 bread roll 1 doughnut	work	* * *		Bought more food from canteen. Shouldn't have eaten the egg sandwich – too much.
3.45	1 doughnut 1 cup tea 1 danish pastry	work	* * *		Bound to be a terrible day now. Can't stop eating. Help.
4.00	2 cups of tea	work		V	Weighed myself – 9st. 4lbs. Cried MUST NOT EAT AGAIN TODAY.
8.20	1 slice of toast 1 slice of toast	kitchen	* *		Lonely, bored. I need someone to talk to.
8.35	1 slice of toast 1 diet coke	kitchen	*		
8.40	Whole packet of shortbread biscuits	kitchen	*		Give up. I can't go on like this. Hate myself.
8.52	1 bowl of cereal 2 glasses of water		*		
9.05	1 bowl of cereal		*	V	Feel completely bloated. Weighed 9st. 5lbs. Wish I was dead.
				L	– 16 Nylax

B, bulimic episodes; V/P, vomiting or purgative use; L, laxative use; * episodes of eating viewed by the patient as 'excessive'

Source: 'Assessment of the specific psychopathology of bulimia nervosa' by C. G. Fairburn, J. Steere and P. J. Cooper, in M. M. Fitcher (ed.) *Bulimia nervosa: Basic research, diagnosis & therapy*. Copyright 1990 John Wiley & Sons Limited. Reproduced with permission

C: Everybody.

T: Suppose it is true that everybody doesn't like you, what then?

C: I must be liked; I must not be rejected by people.

T: What will it mean to you if you are not liked and are rejected by people?

C: That will be terrible and I am no good and unlovable then.

(Lam, 2001, p. 4)[1]

This excerpt provides some insight into Rachel's thinking and, as Lam (2001) pointed out, her need to have dietary control seemed to be related to concerns about self-worth and the belief that she would be rejected, and may also have been tied in with her perfectionism. Fairburn (1997, p. 212) has also argued that many bulimics tend to be perfectionist by nature.

Atypical eating disorders

In the NCCMH guidelines, atypical eating disorders are defined as 'Eating disorders of clinical severity that do not meet the diagnostic criteria of anorexia nervosa or bulimia nervosa'. The equivalent American term is 'eating disorder not otherwise specified' ('EDNOS') (American Psychiatric Association (APA), 1994). The terms apply to eating disorders that are similar to anorexia and bulimia but do not meet the necessary diagnostic criteria. It could be that an atypical eating disordered person's weight is just above the threshold for anorexia, menstruation may not have ceased, or binge eating and purging behaviour may occur less frequently than is usually accepted for the diagnosis of bulimia. As in anorexia and bulimia, there is often an over-concern with body weight and shape and keeping strict control of food intake. This form of eating disorder can be as severe and long lasting as anorexia and bulimia, with the person involved often feeling distressed and upset about the binges and avoiding social interaction (NCCMH, 2004).

This category also includes binge eating disorder (BED), which, like bulimia, includes people who take part in uncontrollable episodes of binge eating. However, unlike bulimia, the individuals concerned do not purge or use other compensatory behaviour afterwards. According to the NCCMH guidelines (2004), the characteristics of binge eating disorder can include eating much more rapidly than normal, eating until feeling uncomfortably full, eating large amounts of food when not physically hungry, eating alone through embarrassment at the amount one is eating, feeling disgust or extreme guilt after overeating.

Epstein (1993) describes the case of Carole, a compulsive overeater. Carole would buy large amounts of food and consume it on her way home from work, or eat indiscriminately from the food that she had in her kitchen. Carole binged to offset unpleasant moods and emotions and described food as a 'drug', which links the discussion here to propositions outlined in Brown's (1997) model:

I would often binge on an evening or a weekend when I had nothing to do, so that I would not feel lonely. I ate to relieve stress, boredom, anxiety . . . I never ate when I was happy . . . Before I joined overeaters anonymous, I craved food every 10 minutes. Food was a drug that had stopped working for me. It no longer made me feel better. I would eat so much at night that I could not get up to be at work on time, and I desperately needed my job.

(Epstein, 1993, pp. 71–2)

It should be stated that some authors have been critical of the DSM-IV category EDNOS and, by extension, atypical eating disorders. Palmer (2005; see also Moor *et al.*, 2004) in particular has set out a number of problems associated with EDNOS, stating that:

The classification of the eating disorders achieves the standard of being collectively exhaustive only through having the 'rag bag' or residual category of EDNOS. The EDNOS category has only one positive criterion and one negative criterion. The positive criterion is that the individual being thus diagnosed should be deemed to have an eating disorder of clinical severity – a disorder that matters. The negative criterion is that the disorder should not fulfil criteria for AN [anorexia nervosa] or BN [bulimia nervosa].

(Palmer, 2005, p. 3)

For Palmer (2005), the limitation of its two criteria, one of which, the positive criterion, is not defined, is a major weakness of the EDNOS category. He asks 'Where is the line to be drawn that defines a state as an *eating* disorder and of *clinical* significance?' It is important to keep these problems in mind as, according to Palmer, EDNOS is the most common diagnosis among people presenting to eating disorder services.

Recognizing eating disorders

Clinical diagnosis

Diagnosis is usually made on the basis of a comprehensive assessment that often examines current and past physical health and treatment, cognitive capacities, physical disabilities, historical and current family and interpersonal relationships, mental state and personality, social circumstances and supports, occupational and social functioning, and education and vocational needs (NCCMH, 2004). A second, corroborative account from a relative or friend about these aspects of a client's history can prove useful because anorexics and bulimics tend to be secretive about their behaviour. During an assessment, therefore, clients may be reluctant or ambivalent about providing accurate information. The perception that, in any treatment, they may be prevented from engaging in restricted food intake, or bingeing and compensatory behaviour, may increase their fears about excessive weight gain and make them reluctant to cooperate.

Physical examinations are very important for assessing the physical impact of eating disorders. These include basic weight and height measurement and calculation of BMI. For adults with anorexia, a BMI below, and with bulimia, a BMI above 17.5 kg/m² is considered the cut-off point. Further medical tests may involve haematological tests, electrocardiography, radiological assessment and ultrasound. Where possible, clinical observation can also allow the characteristics of eating disorder behaviours to be observed (NCCMH, 2004).

In formulating its guidelines for diagnosis of eating disorders, the NCCMH (2004) incorporated diagnostic criteria from both the American Psychiatric Association's *Diagnostic and Statistical Manual*, 4th edition (1994; DSM–IV) and the 10th edition of the *International Classification of Diseases* published by the World Health Organization (ICD10; WHO, 1992).

Anorexia athletica

The term *anorexia athletica* is often used in the sport psychology literature as a term for an eating disorder condition that is found among athletes (e.g. Beals, 2004; Thompson and Sherman, 1993). It seems it was first used by Pugliese *et al.* (1983) and later picked up by others, especially Sundgot-Borgen (e.g. 1993, 1994a, 1994b) who modified it in her work on eating disorders in elite Norwegian athletes. Anorexia athletica is the label given to a category used to classify athletes who do not meet the DSM-III-R (APA, 1987) criteria for anorexia, bulimia or EDNOS, but who show symptoms of a sub-clinical eating disorder. Some of the symptoms of anorexia athletica are similar to those of anorexia and bulimia, including a fear of gaining weight, reduction in food intake and, often, the use of vomiting, laxatives and/or diuretics to offset planned binge eating. To meet the criteria for anorexia athletica, female sports performers must weigh 5 per cent or more below the normal weight for females of the same age and height in the general population; have gastrointestinal complaints; have weight reduction that can not be explained by any medical illness or affective disorder; have an excessive fear of becoming obese; have reduced their food intake through, for example, dieting to less than 1,200 calories per day. In addition, there are several relative criteria that are also thought to be important for diagnosing the condition. These are: delayed puberty; menstrual dysfunction; disturbed body image; use of purging; binge eating and compulsive exercise.

These criteria are very similar to the NCCMH (2004) criteria for anorexia and bulimia nervosa. Currently, anorexia athletica is not recognized in the NCCMH guidelines or in the DSM-III-R (APA, 1987) or DSM-IV (APA, 1994) as a sub-clinical condition. Time will tell whether this extra label and category of eating disorder problems will prove of real benefit to the understanding of eating disorders in athletes. More information on eating disorders in athletes will be presented in the following chapter.

Assessment through self-report inventories

In addition to diagnostic criteria, questionnaire measures have been developed to assess the presence of disordered eating. Self-report eating disorder inventories are dependent on respondents honestly and accurately describing their symptoms. However, the tendency for individuals with eating disorders to be secretive about their behaviour and, especially for anorexics, to deny that they have a serious problem (Garner and Garfinkel, 1979; Kashubeck-West et al., 2001) may affect test scores, although Garner and Garfinkel (1979) claimed that it did not prevent the identification of patients with anorexia in their test results. Comprehensive reviews of eating disorder self-report inventories can be found elsewhere (e.g. Allison, 1995; Kashubeck-West et al., 2001). Two of the most commonly used self-report inventories in the eating disorder literature are described here. These are the Eating Attitudes Test (EAT) (Garner and Garfinkel, 1979) and the Eating Disorder Inventory (EDI) (Garner and Olmsted, 1984; Garner et al., 1983) and, to illustrate their usefulness, example studies using each measure are also described. These studies were deliberately chosen because they also involve exercise and the results help to clarify the link between eating disorders and exercise.

The Eating Attitudes Test (EAT) was one of the first instruments designed to measure symptoms of anorexia nervosa. It is a 40-item, 6-point Likert-type scale and a total score of 30 or above is considered indicative of an eating disorder. Later, Garner et al. (1982) developed a shortened 26-item version based on a factor analysis of the original EAT scale. The tests were highly correlated with each other (correlation coefficient $r = 0.98$) and became known as EAT-40 And EAT-26, respectively. However, as changes to the DSM criteria have been made since the development of these tests, it has become apparent that, while many of the items are associated with anorexic attitudes and behaviour, other items are associated more with bulimia criteria and symptoms as defined by the DSM-IV (Kashubeck-West et al., 2001; Mintz and O'Halloran, 2001). Mintz and O'Halloran (2001) found, after reviewing the published psychometric EAT data, that both measures had good validity for identifying undifferentiated eating disorders, including anorexia, bulimia and eating disorders not otherwise specified, rather than anorexia as specifically intended by the original authors. Thus, some 25 years after the development of the tests, EAT is not recommended for the screening of specific eating disorders, as individuals scoring above 30 for the EAT-40 cut-off and 20 for the EAT-26 cut-off are likely to include individuals with different types of eating disorder (Kashubeck-West et al., 2001). However, research using the EAT measure has provided some valuable data on the profiles of those suffering from eating disorders.

For example, the EAT questionnaire was used by Long *et al.* (1993) in their comparison of behaviour and attitudes in anorexic and normal samples. The anorexic group included 21 female anorexics who were in-patients in an eating disorders unit. The 'normal' or control groups consisted of 42 females and 20 males, matched approximately for age in five-year age bands (average age for each of the anorexic, male control and female control groups was 25 years). Participants were screened for anorexia and two potential participants, identified as former anorexics, were excluded. All participants completed two questionnaires about their exercise behaviour and attitudes and a slightly modified version of the Commitment to Running Questionnaire (CRQ) (Carmack and Martens, 1979) that was used as a measure of positive addiction to exercise (Glasser, 1976). In addition, anorexics completed the EAT measure, the Culture Free Self-Esteem Inventory (SEI) (Battle, 1981) and the Brief Symptom Inventory (BSI) (Derogatis and Spencer, 1982).

A number of interesting results were obtained. Anorexics took part in significantly more exercise activities per week than the normal groups. For those who exercised on a daily basis, the majority of non-clinical controls (60 per cent) exercised for 15–20 minutes while the majority of anorexics (63 per cent) exercised for over 30 minutes per day. The only participants who exercised for more than an hour per day were from the anorexia group (29 per cent). Solitary or secretive exercise was more likely in anorexics and this was correlated significantly with low self-esteem (SEI), depression, anxiety, and phobic anxiety (all BSI). Long *et al.* (1993) argued that this result reflected the social withdrawal that is typical of anorexia as the condition progresses and as the amount of exercise increases. The anorexic group was also more hyperactive than control participants, a result that supported previous reports (e.g. Kron *et al.*, 1978).

Responses indicated that if they were sick or injured, all of the anorexic daily exercisers continued to exercise and, if prevented from exercising, experienced withdrawal symptoms, including anxiety, guilt or depression. Exercise was significantly more likely to be used by female anorexics than by normal males for weight control and significantly more likely to be used to cope with negative emotional states by anorexics than by the control groups. Long *et al.* (1993) concluded that anorexics may need excessive amounts of exercise to produce a positive mood change because starvation increases the experience of negative mood states. In addition, anorexics were found to be more compulsive about exercise and spend more time thinking about it than normal participants.

Among the anorexia group, the main motives for exercise were concerned with controlling negative affect, counteracting the fear of not being able to exercise, and possibly avoiding withdrawal effects (Long *et al.*, 1993). Since the initial motive for exercise among anorexics was thought to be for fitness purposes (Touyz *et al.*, 1987), Long *et al.*'s (1993) results appeared to indicate that the motives of anorexics for exercise may change as weight is reduced. Finally, even though no important differences between groups were found in positive addiction scores using the CRQ, significantly more anorexics than normals showed negative addiction to exercise, suggesting that this behaviour is a true negative addiction with little positive benefit.

The Eating Disorder Inventory (EDI) (Garner and Olmsted, 1984; Garner et al., 1983) was designed to assess psychological and behavioural dimensions common in anorexia and bulimia. There are eight subscales comprising 64 individual items each with a 6-point Likert-type scale. The eight subscales are: *drive for thinness, bulimia, body dissatisfaction, ineffectiveness, perfectionism, interpersonal distrust, interoceptive awareness* and *maturity fears*. Subscale scores can be totalled or considered individually. A total score of 42 is considered indicative of an eating disorder. The first three subscales of the measure assess attitudes and behaviours related to eating, weight and body shape, and the latter five measure features that have been identified as aspects of the psychopathology of anorexia nervosa (Davis, 1990). A second measure, the Eating Disorder Inventory 2 (EDI-2) was published by Garner (1991). This instrument included the original 64 items plus another 27 'provisional' items grouped into three provisional subscales: *asceticism, impulse regulation* and *social insecurity*. However, the original EDI has been used much more frequently in the exercise and sport literature than EDI-2. In reviewing research that has used the EDI, Kashubeck-West et al. (2001) pointed out that, while the EDI appears to have good test-retest reliability, research findings are contradictory when it has been used to discriminate between subgroups of anorexics and bulimics, as different studies found different groups to have higher scores. The EDI has low specificity and, because several of the subscales are concerned with general psychological disturbance, it can be difficult to separate people with eating disorders from those with other psychological disorders. For these reasons, some caution is required when using the instrument for research or counselling practice (Kashubeck-West et al., 2001).

In a good example of research using the EDI and exercise, Davis (1990) examined the relationships between addictive personality traits, weight and diet preoccupation, and exercise participation in a non-clinical population. Ninety-six women volunteers, whose average age was 26 years, were divided into two groups of exercisers and non-exercisers on the basis of the frequency and duration of their participation in physical exercise activities (e.g. running, swimming, cycling, aerobics classes). Their height and weight were measured and Body Mass Index calculated. They also completed the EDI and the Eysenck Personality Questionaire (EPQ) (Eysenck and Eysenck, 1975). The EPQ measures four personality dimensions (*extraversion, neuroticism, psychoticism* and *social desirability*) and provides a measure of *addictiveness*. The findings indicated that in exercisers, but not in non-exercisers, *addictiveness* was positively and significantly related to all the weight and diet variables, including *drive for thinness, body dissatisfaction, bulimia* and *weight and diet preoccupation*. Exercisers were also found to place a significantly greater emphasis on the *importance of their appearance* and scored significantly lower on *psychoticism* than non-exercisers. Finally, *perfectionism* and *addictiveness* were found to be positively related in exercisers, but not in non-exercisers. Davis (1990) advanced a number of possible explanations for these results, but argued that the most feasible was that women with a strong body focus are more likely to exercise regularly, and those with addictive personality characteristics in this group tend to become more preoccupied with dieting and more critical of their appearance than the others. She also argued that, for certain susceptible women, physical activity may not just be a consequence of preoccupation with weight, but it may play a central and antecedent role in its development in some women.

In an earlier related study, de Silva and Eysenck (1987) also used the EPQ and found that addiction scale scores for bulimics were significantly higher than those for anorexics. Bulimics' addictiveness scores were found to be almost as high as those for drug addicts and very different from those of normal participants. Bulimics' and drug addicts' overall personality profiles (low *extraversion*, high *neuroticism* and elevated *psychoticism*) were very similar. This led the researchers to conclude from their results that bulimia may be best seen as a form of addiction (see also Davis and Claridge, 1998). In this respect, it is interesting to note that both Orford (2001) and Brown (1997) included eating in their models of the so-called 'core addictions' (see Chapter 2). The following section examines bulimia and anorexia in more detail from the point of view of aspects of Brown's (1997) model and reversal theory (Brown, 1988, 2001).

Eating disorders, Brown's Hedonic Management Model and reversal theory

In Chapter 2, arguments were presented and research evidence reviewed to establish the proposition that certain activities, such as gambling and drinking alcohol, could be used by individuals to manipulate felt arousal levels and positively influence hedonic tone. This proposition forms a central feature of Brown's (1997) Hedonic Management Model of Addictions and his addition of reversal theory formulations (Brown, 1988, 2001). Many of those with eating problems also use eating, or refraining from eating, in a similar way, as a means of manipulating arousal levels and, through them, hedonic tone (Kerr, Frank-Regan and Brown, 1993).

Kerr *et al.* (1993), in their theory paper, discussed eating disorders mostly from the point of view of reversal theory's telic and paratelic states. The next section of this chapter will include the main thrust of their arguments but also extend the discussion to include other concepts from the theory that might play a role in the explanation of eating disorders. The discussion will first examine bulimia, which most closely follows the felt arousal and hedonic tone 'roller coaster' that Brown (1988) described for the gambler, and then move on to consider anorexic behaviour as a dependency or addiction.

Bulimia

Bulimics often engage in planned episodes of binge eating of large amounts of food when experiencing anxiety, depression or tension (e.g. Cooper and Bowskill, 1986; NCCMH, 2004). Planning and executing the binge episode represents an arousal-raising enterprise that can relieve the anhedonia felt by the bulimic (Brown, 1997; Kerr *et al.*, 1993). For them, the planning necessary for the binge (buying or assembling food and planning for an uninterrupted eating session) and, for example, the experience of anxiety prior to a binge are likely to take place in a telic-conformist state combination with accompanying unpleasant high arousal. During binges, the experience of unpleasant feelings is often changed into a highly pleasant experience, which may even take the form of 'feverish excitement' (Wijesinghe, 1977). These feelings of (feverish) excitement during the binge suggest that the attempt to achieve (very) high levels of arousal through binge eating have been successful. This successful transition would have been facilitated by a telic to paratelic and conformist to negativistic state reversals that allowed high arousal to be reinterpreted as pleasant excitement and high levels of felt negativism to be enjoyed, as a self-imposed rule not to eat is broken. It is also likely that the autic and sympathy states would be operative as the person loses the control associated with autic-mastery metamotivation and succumbs to treating and gratifying him or herself with large amounts of food.

An individual's physical capacity for ingesting food would limit his or her ability to maintain the paratelic 'high' and, as the binge episode ends and the person feels tired and sick, reversals back to the telic and conformist states would be likely. In these states, as levels of felt negativism decrease rapidly, high arousal levels would once again be interpreted as unpleasant anxiety. After a binge episode, the bulimic feels self-loathing or self-disgust at having succumbed to the bingeing. In reversal theory terms, all this would suggest that a particular alliance of somatic and transactional states was operative after a binge episode. This alliance would likely involve a telic-conformist and an autic-mastery state combination under conditions of unpleasant high felt arousal and unpleasant low felt transactional outcome. In this case, the 'transaction' concerns the bulimic 'interacting' with him or herself, cognitively evaluating his or her own binge behaviour as reprehensible.

With the telic state likely to be salient after the binge, the adoption and speedy achievement of the new goals of compensatory behaviour in the form of vomiting and purging make possible the resumption of eating. The sight of food may then bring about reversals to the paratelic and negativistic states, in which high arousal and high felt negativism can again be enjoyed. After several cycles of such reversals, the binge episode is likely to be limited only by the onset of exhaustion or by the food running out. Should either of these eventualities occur, and as the relatively short-term positive effects of binge eating dissipate, the individual is again likely to be in the intensely anhedonic metamotivational pattern described above.

In this somewhat simplified reversal theory view of bulimic binge episodes, it is likely that some other reversals and/or variations in felt arousal, negativism and transactional outcome levels would occur over time within any series of binge eating and compensatory activity (purging, vomiting, abstinence or exercise). For example, it is unlikely that during such a series of binge eating episodes felt arousal could be maintained at a high level throughout. It is likely that dominance could also play a role; for example, as Kerr *et al.* (1993) speculated, the more paratelic dominant bulimics are, the more pronounced their bulimia is likely to be.

Popkess-Vawter and her colleagues (e.g. Popkess-Vawter *et al.*, 1998; Popkess-Vawter *et al.*, 2000) have provided research evidence that provides some support for this reversal theory-informed analysis of bulimic behaviour. Their work focused on obese individuals and their overeating behaviour and found that incidents of bingeing and overeating were associated with *overeating tension*, which is the basic assumption behind the reversal theory-based Overeating Tension Scale (OTS) (Popkess-Vawter *et al.*, 2000). Overeating tension is defined as the total discrepancy score resulting from differences between participants' ratings of actual and desired feelings before overeating and concerns tension in relation to all four pairs of motivational states. For example, as in the reversal theory description of the bulimic behaviour above, the overeater experiencing high arousal in the telic state is subject to a degree of tension, or *tension stress* as it has been termed elsewhere (Svebak, 1997), and uses binge eating to decrease the feelings of tension by inducing a reversal to the paratelic state and allowing the high arousal to be enjoyed. In reversal theory, the presence of overeating tension, or tension stress, is reflected in the individual's experience of unpleasant emotions (e.g. anxiety, boredom, resentment, shame and guilt).

Anorexia

The anorexic is typically completely preoccupied with thoughts of food and eating but determined never to give in to the impulse to eat, and dominated by the need to have control over his or her body. It is likely that the anorexic is telic dominant, perhaps at the extreme of telic dominance and subject to persistent telic-conformist and autic-mastery state combinations. As the anorexic becomes more and more truly hungry, the images of food also produce a sense of striving, anxiety and deprivation and so help to maintain this persistent state combination with perhaps the telic state salient. Almost any reversal to the paratelic (and possibly negativistic) state at this stage could result in a bulimic binge, as occurs with many anorexics (Kerr *et al.*, 1993). Recent research results from anorexics in France (Cardenal, 2003), correspond exactly with this theoretical analysis. The results have provided a clear picture of the telic, conformist, autic and mastery basis of the problem.

However, while it is clear from the descriptions above that the bulimic is 'hooked on' paratelic-negativistic-oriented highs associated with binge episodes, in a way that fits well with Brown's (1997) model of addictions, the psychological pattern for the anorexic is different to some extent. It is known that anorexics often experience prolonged negative moods and emotions such as anxiety and depression and feelings of low self-esteem and self-confidence (APA, 1994; NCCMH, 2004). Given this negative psychological experience, the anorexic uses extreme dieting with very limited food intake to maintain tight control over body weight and shape, in an attempt to offset these unpleasant feelings. As a result of sticking to (telic-conformist-based) limited eating goals, the anorexic feels pleasure and satisfaction on achieving them. Decreases in anxiety and depression and lower levels of unpleasant felt arousal follow this positive achievement. The improved emotional tone for the somatic states is augmented by another source of positive hedonic tone arising from the transactional states. The feeling of being in control, positive comments from important others about the anorexic's slim body – at least in the early stages (Lauren, 2005) – and/or self-perceptions (likely short-lived) about looking less fat and having become thinner, lead to positive levels of felt transactional outcome and the experience of pride in the autic and mastery states: 'I wasn't really bothered about getting any help for my anorexia. I felt as if I didn't need help at that time. I felt great, after all' (Hague, 1987, p. 11).

Thus, as it may be the only way for the anorexic to off-set unpleasant feelings, over time the anorexic becomes dependent on this overall improved hedonic tone and continues with restricted food consumption and dieting as a means of achieving it. The strong reinforcement that results from improvements in overall hedonic tone through tight control of eating acts as a crucial factor in the development of a full-blown addiction (Brown, 1997). As reinforcement and positive feedback loops become established, they make it more likely that the increasingly salient behaviour will continue as one of the few sources, or perhaps even the sole source of reward in the anorexic's life. The situation is further complicated by the fact that anhedonia increases with starvation. The consequences may eventually prove to be fatal, as Kerr *et al.* (1993), referring to the final stages of anorexia, pointed out:

> As starvation and emaciation progress, there are physical effects with psychological sequelae. The images of food become more unreal and the feelings of hunger diminish. It is possible that in the terminal stages of anorexia, a reversal to the paratelic state may thus ensue. In this state, perhaps vouchsafed to the dying anorectic, all thoughts and perceptions are bounded by a secure frame of unreality. The former constant telic striving and the unpleasant high arousal have been banished for ever and give way to a pure form of enjoyment of the here and now.
>
> (Kerr *et al.*, 1993, pp. 78–9)

Bulimia and anorexia are conditions that are similar to other reversal-based pathological conditions (Lafreniere *et al.*, 2001). In this sense, individuals with anorexia or bulimia are subject to the type of imbalance and rigidity in metamotivational states and reversals described by Miller (1985), or reversal inhibition described by Apter (1989/2006). This means that the individuals concerned are often stuck in persistent metamotivational state combinations with only occasional reversals to other states. Long *et al.* (1993) provided some support for the reversal theory standpoint in their research findings with anorexic patients. Examining their results in reversal theory terms, it appears that, as starvation continues, it locks the anorexic deeper and deeper into a state of anhedonia. This requires greater and greater amounts of exercise to induce necessary reversals that allow brief periods of positive mood experience.

Closing comments

Within the material on anorexia and bulimia presented in this chapter, including the NCCMH definitions that include exercise, the quotes from people who have suffered from eating disorders, and research findings (e.g. Long *et al.*, 1993), is strong evidence that these conditions are often linked with excessive exercising. In the case of Madelyn, for example, exercise was an integral part of her anorexic condition ('I was up all night exercising') (Epstein, 1993, p. 60), and, in her case and that of many other anorexics, the 'exercise may simply have become another weapon in the arsenal dedicated to rigid weight control' (Garner *et al.*, 1985, p. 517, cited in Davis, 1990). This is precisely the relationship between eating disorders and exercise encompassed in the notion of secondary exercise dependence detailed in Chapter 1 (De Coverly Veale, 1987; Veale, 1995). However, Long and Smith (1990) provided some words of caution about the nature of the link between exercise and eating disorders, specifically anorexia, which are worth noting here:

> The status of excessive activity in anorexia nervosa remains unclear since different investigators view it as a prodromal feature of the disorder (Kron *et al.*, 1978), as a behavioural symptom and as a risk factor for relapse given its tendency to persist after weight restoration. However, a significant number of anorexic patients are not hyperactive. Not all individuals who exercise compulsively are anorexic or become so despite a higher than normal incidence of eating disorders in athletes (Pasman and Thompson, 1988). Further, not all individuals with anorexia nervosa who are excessively active have been premorbidly so, although it may be speculated that the persistence of the behaviour after weight restoration is more likely in those individuals where overactivity provides one of the setting conditions for the disorder.
>
> (Long and Smith, 1990, p. 302)

Also, as Davis (1990) stated:

> it may not be appropriate to consider physical activity merely as a
> consequence of weight preoccupation, but to consider the possibility
> that it may play, for certain susceptible women, a central and antecedent
> role in its development. The widely acclaimed health benefits of regular
> physical activity also contain the subtle message that the pursuit of
> good health should be the pursuit of *ultra-slenderness*. Exercise adherence,
> therefore, can offer intrinsic incentives for some women to embark on
> a cycle of dieting and weight preoccupation in their efforts to achieve
> the elusive ideal.
>
> (Davis, 1990, p. 826)

Extrapolating further, the relationship between eating disorders and exercise
may not be as straightforward as it might first appear. Both Long and Smith
(1990) and Davis (1990) seem to be arguing that not only may exercise be
used as part of rigid weight control, but excessive exercising may also lead
to the development of eating disorders. Sundgot-Borgen (1994a, 1994b)
reported results obtained in a series of studies by Epling and Pierce (1988)
and Epling *et al.* (1983) that led these authors to suggest that as many as
75 per cent of the cases of anorexia nervosa are exercise-induced. Although
at face value this figure appears to be high, they argued that strenuous exercise
tends to suppress appetite, which then decreases the reinforcing value of
food and thus decreases food intake. As body weight decreases with less
food intake, the individual's motivation for higher levels of exercise increases.
If these arguments about exercise-induced eating disorders are correct, then
it is possible that there are two types of dependence involving exercise and
eating disorders: that proposed by Veale (De Coverly Veale, 1987; Veale
1995) where exercise dependence is secondary to an eating disorder; and
one where the eating disorder is secondary to exercise dependence. While
this second type is a possibility, it would require clinical case evidence and
more research findings before it could be considered acceptable as a bona
fide clinical condition.

Finally, in the Long and Smith (1990) quote above, reference is made to
research work that showed a higher than normal incidence of eating disorders
in athletes (Pasman and Thompson, 1988). Almost thirty years after this
publication appeared, it is now well recognized in sport psychology that
athletes in certain types of sports are at risk for developing eating disorders.
This issue is addressed in the following chapter, which takes a comprehensive
look at athletes and eating disorders, identifying the sports in which athletes
are most susceptible to eating disorders and discussing how and why these
might develop.

Notes

1 Source: 'Cognitive behaviour therapy to treating bulimia nervosa: A case study', by D. Lam, *Counselling Psychology Quarterly* (2001) Vol. 14, pp. 1–13. Copyright Taylor and Francis Ltd.: www.tandf.co.uk/journals. Reproduced with permission.

References

Allison, D. B. (1995) *Handbook of assessment methods for eating behaviors and weight-related problems: Measures, theory and research*, Thousand Oaks CA: Sage.

American Psychiatric Association (APA) (1987) *Diagnostic and statistical manual of mental disorders* (3rd edition – revised) (DSM-III-R), Washington DC: American Psychiatric Association.

American Psychiatric Association (APA) (1994) *Diagnostic and statistical manual of mental disorders* (4th edition) Washington DC: American Psychiatric Association.

Apter, M. J. (1989) *Reversal theory: Motivation, emotion and personality*, London: Routledge. (2nd edition published 2006.)

Apter, M. J. (2006) *Reversal theory: The dynamics of motivation, emotion and personality*, 2nd edition, Oxford: Oneworld Publications.

Battle, J. (1981) *A Culture Free Self-Esteem Inventory*, Windsor: Nelson.

Beals, K. A. (2004) *Disordered eating among athletes*, Champaign, IL: Human Kinetics.

Brown, R. I. F. (1988) 'Reversal theory and subjective experience in the explanation of addiction and relapse', in M. J. Apter, J. H. Kerr and M. P. Cowles (eds) *Progress in reversal theory*, Amsterdam: Elsevier, 191–212.

Brown, R. I. F. (1997) 'A theoretical model of behavioural addictions – Applied to offending', in J. E. Hodge, M. McMurran and C. R. Hollin (eds) *Addicted to crime?*, New York: Wiley, 13–65.

Brown, R. I. F. (2001) 'Addictions', in M. J. Apter (ed.) *Motivational styles in everyday life: A guide to reversal theory*, Washington DC: American Psychological Association, 155–65.

Brownell, K. (1991) 'Dieting and the search for the perfect body: Where physiology and culture collide', *Behavior Therapy*, 22, 1–12.

Cardenal, M. (2003) 'Approche differentielle et psychodynamique du rapport subjectif au risque chez les toxicomanes et les anorexiques restrictives', unpublished PhD thesis, Toulouse: University of Toulouse le Mirail, France.

Carmack, M. A. and Martens, R. (1979) 'Measuring commitment to running. A survey of runners' attitudes and mental states', *Journal of Sport Psychology*, 1, 25–42.

Cooper, M. (2003) *The psychology of bulimia nervosa: A cognitive perspective*, Oxford: Oxford University Press.

Cooper, P. J. and Bowskill, R. (1986) 'Dysphoric mood and overeating', *British Journal of Clinical Psychology*, 25, 155–6.

Davis, C. (1990) 'Weight and diet preoccupation and addictiveness: The role of exercise', *Personality and Individual Differences*, 11, 823–7.

Davis, C. and Claridge, D. C. (1998) 'The eating disorders as addiction: A psychobiological perspective', *Addictive Behavior*, 23, 463–75.

Davis, C., Claridge, G. and Fox, J. (2000) 'Not just a pretty face: Physical attractiveness and perfectionism in the risk for eating disorders', *International Journal of Eating Disorders*, 27, 67–73.

De Coverly Veale, D. M. W. (1987) 'Exercise dependence', *British Journal of Addiction*, 82, 735–40.

De Silva, P. and Eysenck, S. (1987) 'Personality and addictiveness in anorexic and bulimic patients', *Personality and Individual Differences*, 8, 749–51.

Derogatis, L. R. and Spencer, T. M. (1982) *The Brief Symptom Inventory: Administration, scoring and procedures manual*. Rider Wood MD: Clinical Psychometric Research.

Epling, W. F. and Pierce, W. D. (1988) 'Activity based anorexia nervosa', *International Journal of Eating Disorders*, 7, 475–85.

Epling, W. F., Pierce, W. D. and Stefan, L. (1983) 'A theory of activity based anorexia', *International Journal of Eating Disorders*, 3, 27–46.

Epstein, R. (1993) *Eating habits and disorders*, New York: Chelsea House Publishers.

Eysenck, H. J. and Eysenck, S. B. G. (1975) *Manual of the Eysenck Personality Questionnaire*, London: Hodder & Stoughton.

Fairburn, C. G. (1997) 'Eating disorders', in D. M. Clark and C. G. Fairburn (eds) *Science and practice of cognitive behaviour therapy*, Oxford: Oxford University Press.

Fairburn, C. G. and Beglin, S. J. (1990) 'Studies on the epidemiology of bulimia nervosa', *American Journal of Psychiatry*, 147, 401–8.

Fairburn, C. G., Steere, J. and Cooper, P. J. (1990) 'Assessment of the specific psychopathology of bulimia nervosa', in M. M. Fitcher (ed.) *Bulimia nervosa: Basic research, diagnosis & therapy*, Chichester: Wiley, 37–57.

Garner, D. M. (1991) *Eating Disorder Inventory-2 professional manual*, Odessa FL: Psychological Assessment Resources.

Garner, D. M. and Garfinkel, P. E. (1979) 'The Eating Attitudes Test: An index of the symptoms of anorexia nervosa', *Psychological Medicine*, 9, 273–9.

Garner, D. M. and Olmsted, M. P. (1984) *Eating Disorder Inventory manual*, Odessa FL: Psychological Assessment Resources.

Garner, D. M., Olmsted, M. P., Bohr, Y. and Garfinkel, P. E. (1982) 'The Eating Attitudes Test: Psychometric features and clinical correlates', *Psychological Medicine*, 12, 871–8.

Garner, D. M., Olmsted, M. P. and Polivy, J. (1983) 'Development and validation of a multi-dimensional Eating Disorder Inventory for anorexia nervosa and bulimia', *International Journal of Eating Disorders*, 2, 15–34.

Garner, D. M., Rockert, W., Olmsted, M. P., Johnson, C. and Coscina, D. V. (1985) 'Psychological principles in the treatment of bulimia and anorexia nervosa', in D. M. Garner and P. E. Garfinkel (eds) *Handbook for psychotherapy for anorexic nervosa and bulimia*, New York: Guildford Press (cited in Davis, C., 1990).

Glasser, W. (1976) *Positive addiction*, New York: Harper & Row.

Hague, D. (1987) 'Pull yourself together, girl', *The Guardian*, 21 November, 11.

Herzog, D. B., Keller, M. B., Sacks, N. R., Yeh, C. J. and Lavori, P. W. (1992) 'Psychiatric comorbidity in treatment-seeking anorexics and bulimics', *Journal of the American Academy of Child and Adolescent Psychiatry*, 31, 810–17.

Kashubeck-West, S., Mintz, L. B. and Saunders, K. J. (2001) 'Assessment of eating disorders in women', *The Counseling Psychologist*, 29, 662–94.

Kerr, J. H., Frank-Regan, E. and Brown, R. I. F. (1993) 'Taking risks with health', *Patient Education and Counseling*, 22, 73–80.

Kron, L., Katz, J. L., Gorzynski, G. and Viner, H. (1978) 'Hyperactivity in anorexia nervosa: A fundamental clinical feature', *Comprehensive Psychiatry*, 19, 432–9.

Lafreniere, K. D., Ledgerwood, D. M. and Murgatroyd, S. J. (2001) 'Psychopathology, therapy and counseling', in M. J. Apter (ed.) *Motivational styles in everyday life: A guide to reversal theory*, Washington DC: American Psychological Association, 263–85.

Lam, D. (2001) 'Cognitive behaviour therapy to treating bulimia nervosa: A case study', *Counselling Psychology Quarterly*, 14, 1–13.

Lauren, J. (2005) 'Jenny Lauren: Beauty was my curse', *The Independent*, 10 October. Online. Available http://news.independent.co.uk.

Long, C. and Smith, J. (1990) 'The treatment of compulsive over-exercising in anorexia nervosa: A case study', *Behavioural Psychotherapy*, 18, 295–306.

Long, C., Smith, J., Midgley, M. and Cassidy, T. (1993) 'Over-exercising in anorexic and normal samples: Behavior and attitudes', *Journal of Mental Health*, 2, 321–7.

Lucas, A. R. (2004) *Demystifying anorexia nervosa: An optimistic guide to understanding and healing*, Oxford: Oxford University Press.

Miller, W. R. (1985) 'Addictive behaviour and the theory of psychological reversals', *Addictive Behaviors*, 10, 177–80.

Mintz, L. and O'Halloran, S. E. (2001) 'The Eating Attitudes Test: Validation with DSM-IV eating disorder criteria', *Journal of Personality Assessment*, 74, 489–503.

Moor, S., Vartanian, L. R., Touyz, S. W. and Beumont, P. J. V. (2004) 'Psychopathology of EDNOS patients: To whom do they compare?', *Clinical Psychologist*, 8, 70–5.

National Collaboration Centre for Mental Health (NCCMH) (2004) *Eating disorders*, Leicester: The British Psychological Society and Gaskell.

Orford, J. (2001) *Excessive appetites: A psychological view of addictions*, Chichester: John Wiley.

Palmer, B. (2005) 'Concepts of eating disorders', in J. Treasure, U. Schmidt and E. van Furth (eds) *The essential handbook of eating disorders*, Chichester: John Wiley, 1–10.

Pasman, L. and Thompson, K. (1988) 'Body image and caring disturbance in obligatory runners, obligatory weight lifters, and sedentary individuals', *International Journal of Eating Disorders*, 7, 759–70.

Popkess-Vawter, S., Bandau, C. and Straub, J. (1998) 'Unpleasant emotional triggers to overeating and related intervention strategies for overweight and obese women weight cyclers', *Applied Nursing Research*, 11, 69–76.

Popkess-Vawter, S., Gerkovich, M. M. and Wendel, S. (2000) 'Reliability and validity of the Overeating Tension Scale', *Journal of Nursing Measurement*, 8, 145–59.

Pugliese, M. T., Lifshitz, F., Grad, G., Fort, P., Marks, M. and Katz, J. L. (1983) 'Fear of obesity: A cause of short stature and delayed puberty', *New England Journal of Medicine*, 309, 513–18.

Shafran, R. and de Silva, P. (2005) 'Cognitive behavioural models', in J. Treasure, U. Schmidt and E. van Furth (eds) *The essential handbook of eating disorders*, Chichester: John Wiley, 35–52.

Sundgot-Borgen, J. (1993) 'Prevalence of eating disorders in female elite athletes', *International Journal of Sport Nutrition*, 3, 29–40.

Sundgot-Borgen, J. (1994a) 'Eating disorders in female athletes', *Sports Medicine*, 17, 176–88.

Sundgot-Borgen, J. (1994b) 'Risk and trigger factors for the development of eating disorders in female elite athletes', *Medicine and Science in Sports and Exercise*, 26, 414–19.

Svebak, S. (1997) 'Tension- and effort-stress as predictors of academic performance', in S. Svebak and M. J. Apter (eds), *Stress and health: A reversal theory perspective*, Washington DC: Taylor & Francis, 45–55.

Thompson, R. A., and Sherman, R. T. (1993) *Helping athletes with eating disorders*, Champaign IL: Human Kinetics.

Touyz, S. W., Beumont, T. and Hook, S. (1987) 'Exercise anorexia: A new dimension in anorexia nervosa?', in P. J. V. Beumont, G. D. Burrows and R. C. Caspar (eds) *Handbook of eating disorders Part 1*, New York: Elsevier Science.

Van Hoeken, D., Seidell, J. and Hoek, H. W. (2005) 'Epidemiology', in J. Treasure, U. Schmidt and E. van Furth (eds) *The essential handbook of eating disorders*, Chichester: John Wiley, 10–34.

Veale, D. (1995) 'Does primary exercise dependence really exist?', in J. Annett, B. Cripps and H. Steinberg (eds) *Exercise addiction: Motivation for participation in sport and exercise*, Leicester: The British Psychological Society, 1–5.

Wijesinghe, B. (1977) 'Massed electric aversion treatment of compulsive eating', in J. Foreyt (ed.) *Behavioral treatments of obesity*, Oxford: Pergamon.

World Health Organization (WHO) (1992) *International classification of diseases*, (10th edition) Geneva: World Health Organization.

5 Getting thin to win
Athletes, eating disorders and exercise dependence

Christy Henrich was the third-ranking female gymnast in the United States in the early 1990s. Like many elite female athletes, winning an international gold medal was her primary ambition and motivation. Henrich, known as 'ET' for 'extra tough', typically undertook a daily practice regime that involved two three-hour practice sessions: one that began at 6.30 a.m. and a second that finished at 10 p.m. In between the practice sessions, she took private school lessons with a tutor, as she had decided to leave high school to concentrate on gymnastics and gain a valued place on the US team. In 1988 she came extremely close to becoming a member of the US Olympic team, just missing out by an incredible 0.118 of a point. In 1990, she was still among the top ten US gymnasts and was working towards the 1992 Olympic team trials, when she was forced to withdraw from a competition because she was too weak to compete. As it turned out, she had developed anorexia and bulimia nervosa to the extent that her body was unable to maintain her gymnastic performance, and her aspirations to reach the top became badly affected. The catalyst that set off her eating disorders occurred in 1988, when a judge at an international competition in Budapest told her that she needed to watch her weight. Eventually, she was forced to give up gymnastics because of her eating disorders, which had taken over her life. In 1994, she stated: 'My life is a horrifying nightmare. It feels like there's a beast inside of me, like a monster. It feels evil' (*Japan Times*, 1994). At the height of her career she weighed 93 pounds (42 kilograms), but once she left gymnastics, her weight often plummeted to 60 pounds (27 kilograms). Tragically, some six years after that comment from the judge in Budapest, she lost her battle with her eating disorders and died from multiple organ failure in 1994, aged 22 (*Japan Times*, 1994; Ryan, 1996).

Christy Henrich died as a direct result of her eating disorders and was probably the first international-level performer to do so, but another US Olympic gymnast, Cathy Rigby, had a close escape. As a 15-year-old, Rigby competed in the 1968 Mexico City Summer Olympics and earned the highest-ever US scores in gymnastics. Later, she went on to win a silver medal on the balance beam at the 1970 World Championships and was a member of the 1972 US Olympic team. In total, she won twelve international gymnastics medals, including eight gold medals. After the 1972 Olympics, she retired from gymnastics and took up an acting career. However, it was only in the early 1980s that she was able to recover from the bulimia nervosa condition that had begun when she was a gymnast. During the time she suffered from bulimia, she was hospitalized twice and almost died from cardiac arrest. She also admitted that over half the American Olympic team in 1972 suffered from similar eating disorders (Ryan, 1996).

In the early 1990s, sport psychologists (and experts in other disciplines) really began to wake up to the problem of eating disorders among athletes. The 1994 death of Christy Henrich, Cathy Rigby's revelations about her own almost fatal experience of eating disorders and the 1996 publication of Joan Ryan's exposé of eating disorders among gymnasts and figure skaters all contributed to increased attention being focused on the topic. Ryan (1996), in particular, illustrated the extremes to which some athletes (often encouraged by their coaches, competition judges and sometimes their parents) are prepared to push themselves in order to achieve their personal performance goals. Her book highlighted a 'dark side' to elite sport in which the combined effects of self-starvation, nutrient deprivation, and extremely rigorous training regimes became apparent.

Does sport place athletes at greater risk for eating disorders?

Two meta-analytic studies of research studies have compared disordered eating behaviour in athletes and non-athletes (Hausenblas and Carron, 1999; Smolak et al., 2000). Smolak et al. (2000) carried out a meta-analysis of 34 different studies and found that college (but not high school) athletes did appear to be somewhat more at risk for eating problems than non-athletes. However, as the authors pointed out, while the difference was significant, it has to be treated with caution because of statistical limitations associated with the effect size. Hausenblas and Carron (1999) found that female and male athletes reported more bulimic and anorexic symptoms compared to males and females from the general population, but, as Haase et al. (2002) pointed out, these studies were only able to demonstrate that disordered eating occurs slightly more frequently in athletes than non-athletes.

The evidence from other studies has yielded mixed results. For example, although Taube and Blinde (1992) did find that athletes were significantly more 'perfectionist' and at risk for bulimia, they had significantly higher self-esteem than non-athletes. Low self-esteem is often a characteristic of those who develop anorexia and bulimia. DiBartolo and Shaffer (2002) found that female athletes exhibited significantly healthier attitudes about themselves, their eating and their body shape than female non-athletes, the opposite of what might have been expected if athletes were at increased risk of developing eating disorders. A study by Fulkerson et al. (1999) revealed no significant differences between athletes and non-athletes in the majority of eating disordered behaviours and attitudes. When differences were found, the athletes had more positive attitudes and behaviours. A more recent study by Sundgot-Borgen *et al.* (2004) found the prevalence of eating disorders to be significantly higher among elite athletes than the general population.

It is possible that, in the studies reviewed here, any potential differences were masked by the researchers grouping athletes from a wide variety of different sports in one large sample. There seems to have been little attention paid to the differences in physical demands and the physiques required for effective performance between different sports. In the DiBartolo and Shaffer (2002) study, for example, cross-country runners were grouped with soccer and field hockey players, and these in turn were also grouped with volleyball, basketball and squash players. As will be shown in the next section, a more sophisticated approach to the grouping of athletes in sports with common characteristics, such as that adopted by Sundgot-Borgen (1993, 1994a, 1994b; see also Sundgot-Borgen *et al.*, 2004), would prove useful in research trying to establish whether athletes in certain sports, such as gymnastics, are more likely to develop eating disorders than those involved in others.

In talking about athletes with anorexia, Beals (2004) pointed out that:

> Individuals with anorexia nervosa are notoriously adept at hiding and finding excuses for their extreme, often bizarre eating and exercising behaviors. For the athlete with anorexia nervosa, the sport setting provides not only an expanded repertoire of rationalizations but also an apparently valid context within which weight loss or low body weight as well as rigid and abnormal eating and exercise habits can be justified (Thompson and Sherman, 1993).
>
> (Beals, 2004, p. 8)

The discussion in the following sections will consist of a detailed examination of eating disorder research in athletes in different types of sports. A particular focus of this discussion will be athletes participating in the so-called 'thin-build', 'aesthetic', 'endurance' and 'weight-dependent' sports, which all tend to emphasize leanness (Beals, 2004; Manore and Thompson, 2000; Sundgot-Borgen, 1993, 1994a, 1994b). Where relevant, case study material and quotes from elite athletes will be used in conjunction with research evidence to build up a realistic picture of eating disorders in competitive sport. Some writers (e.g. Grogan, 1999; Petrie and Rogers, 2001) have pleaded the case for men in general and male athletes in particular to be recognized in the eating disorder literature. As was mentioned in Chapter 4, males are thought to make up approximately 10 per cent of those who present with anorexia and bulimia (APA, 1994; Fairburn and Beglin, 1994), and a book publication has been devoted solely to male eating disorders (Langley, 2006). While it is true that much of the research on athletes and eating disorders has concentrated on females, there are now plenty of case examples and research studies that have shown that male athletes can also be subject to eating disorders. Several of these will be reviewed in this chapter.

Eating disorder research in athletes

Sundgot-Borgen (1993, 1994a, 1994b), in her seminal study, used a three-stage design in which 603 female Norwegian athletes were first screened to ensure that they were elite athletes (qualified for, or a member of recruiting squads for, the national team at junior or senior levels); aged between 12 and 35 years; training at least eight hours a week; and competing at least for the next six months. Those who could not fulfil these criteria were excluded from the study, leaving 522 athletes. These athletes, from 35 different sports, were divided into six groups of sports with common elements. These were *technical, aesthetic, weight-dependent, endurance, ball games* and *power* sports. Of these, aesthetic, weight-dependent and endurance sports emphasize leanness (thin-build) and are sports in which a low body weight provides an advantage in competitive performance. Aesthetic sports are those in which judges rate performances in, for example, gymnastics, springboard diving and figure skating. Weight-dependent sports include combat sports, such as judo, karate and wrestling, where athletes must 'make their weight' to compete in weight divisions. Endurance sports are those where the speed and efficiency of movement are enhanced by low body weight, such as middle and long distance running, rowing, cycling, cross-country skiing and swimming. Technical sports include high and long jumping, golf and sailing; ball games include basketball, soccer and volleyball; and discus, javelin and sprinting are examples of power sports.

In the second stage, the EDI (Garner and Olmsted, 1984; Garner *et al.*, 1983; see Chapter 4) and, specifically, the *drive for thinness* and *body dissatisfaction* subscales were used as a second screen for subjects thought to be at risk for eating disorders. Elevated scores on these two subscales indicate individuals at risk for eating disorders (>15 and >10, respectively). Athlete controls (n = 30) did not have increased scores on these subscales. Following this procedure, in stage three, 103 at-risk athletes and the 30 control group athletes were given clinical interviews using an interview protocol developed by Johnson (1985). Finally, 92 athletes were identified who met the criteria for anorexia, bulimia or anorexia athletica (Sundgot-Borgen, 1993, 1994a, 1994b).

The results indicated that the prevalence of eating disorders was found to be significantly higher in athletes from aesthetic and weight-dependent sports than among those sports where leanness was not thought to be important. Aesthetic and endurance sport athletes were leaner and had a significantly higher training volume than athletes in the other sports groups. Some 35 per cent of the aesthetic sport athletes, 29 per cent of the weight-dependent sport athletes and 20 per cent of the endurance sport athletes met the criteria for an eating disorder. Further analysis indicated that, among the 80 athletes within the endurance sport group, cross-country skiing had the largest number of eating disordered athletes (33 per cent), with middle and long distance running next (27.2 per cent), followed by cycling (20 per cent), swimming (15 per cent) and orienteering (0 per cent) (Sundgot-Borgen, 1993, 1994a, 1994b). In addition, among the eating disordered athletes, the study was able to identify three different categories of factors that might trigger the development of eating disorders (Sundgot-Borgen, 1994b). These were: *prolonged periods of dieting or weight fluctuations* (41 per cent); *traumatic events*, for example, illness or injury to the athlete or family member, new coach, casual comments about weight, relationship problems (48 per cent); and *significant increase in training volume* (11 per cent).

An American study conducted in collaboration with the National College Athletic Association (NCAA) (Johnson *et al.*, 1999) had the potential to extend the results of Sundgot-Borgen's study of female Norwegian athletes to both male and female American athletes. Although the American study did include the *body dissatisfaction, drive for thinness* and *bulimia* subscales from the EDI and many of the same sports, the authors did not group similar sports together in their analysis as had been done in the Norwegian study. However, among a range of results reported by Johnson *et al.* (1999), which mostly concentrated on a comparison of male and female athletes, there were some concerned with individual sports that provided some support for Sundgot-Borgen's (1993,1994a, 1994b) results. For example, when possible eating disorders between sports were examined using the three EDI subscales, female gymnasts scored significantly higher than both female swimmers and female basketball players on the *drive for thinness* subscale. However, using the strict DSM-IV criteria for anorexia and bulimia (APA, 1994), none of the athletes could be diagnosed as anorexic, and only 1.1 per cent of females as bulimic. At a sub-clinical level, 2.85 per cent of females exhibited significant symptoms of anorexia, and 9.2 per cent of females exhibited significant symptoms of bulimia.

As it turned out, Sundgot-Borgen extended her first research study to include both male and female athletes (Sundgot-Borgen *et al.*, 2004). The results of this new study largely confirmed the earlier results for female elite athletes and indicated that the prevalence of eating disorders among male athletes was greater in anti-gravitation sports (e.g. athletics: long, triple and high jump) (22 per cent) than in endurance sports (9 per cent), and ball games (5 per cent). Generally, eating disorders were again found to be more prevalent in the leanness-dependent and weight-dependent sports than in other sports.

There is a possibility that competitive level may be a contributory factor in the development of eating disorders. For example, Sundgot-Borgen's (1993, 1994a, 1994b) Norwegian athletes were elite senior or junior national team members or members of the national recruiting squads. Little research has been done on this topic, but Picard (1999) assessed two levels of competitive athletes (US Division I, II) and non-athletes, using the Eating Attitudes

Test (EAT-26; Garner *et al.*, 1982), the Eating Disorders Inventory-2 (EDI-2; Garner, 1991) and a demographic and health questionnaire. The Division I athletes had significantly higher scores on the EAT and EDI scales, positing a higher preoccupation with thinness, weight and diet, and a morbid fear of fat than the other groups. Picard's (1999) results suggest that athletes at a higher level are more at risk for developing eating disorders than less able athletes and non-athletes. Smolak *et al.* (2000) found that elite athletes were significantly more at risk for developing eating disorders than non-athletes, and athletes in elite 'lean' sports were found to be at especially high risk. However, these results must be treated with caution because of statistical limitations.

In summary, the importance of Sundgot-Borgen's (1993, 1994a, 1994b) findings was that they clarified that thin-build sports, in which leanness is important for appearance or performance, place athletes at particularly high risk of developing eating disorders, and also identified three important types of trigger factors that may initiate eating disorders. Sundgot-Borgen's athletes were all high-level performers, and there is some tentative evidence that suggests that athletes at higher levels are at greater risk of developing eating disorders than those at lower levels (Picard, 1999; Smolak *et al.*, 2000). In the discussion below, thin-build sports are at focus, and each of the three categories of sports (aesthetic, weight-dependent and endurance) will be examined separately and in more detail.

Aesthetic sports

Being lean is important in these sports so that the aesthetic quality of the performance in terms of form and appearance is maximized in the eyes of the judges. It seems that 'appearance thinness' is something that can change over time and there has been a trend in recent years in several of these aesthetic sports for athletes to be smaller and to get thinner and thinner. Quoting some figures from Ryan (1996), Johnson *et al.* (1999) pointed out that:

> Appearance thinness refers to the trend over the last decades to reward thinner athletes in the adjudicated sports such as gymnastics and figure skating. In 1972, the winning female gymnastics team had an average height of 5ft 3ins. and an average weight of 106lb. In 1992, the average height was 4ft 9ins and the average weight was 83lb (Ryan, 1995). It is our belief that this trend towards rewarding leanness has contributed to the female athlete's drive for thinness.
>
> (Johnson *et al.*, 1999, p. 187)

In this regard, Zucker *et al.* (1999) compared female college athletes from 'judged' and 'non-judged' sports and regular female students. They held structured interviews and handed out self-report questionnaires to assess the presence of eating disorders, the presence of body weight concerns, psychopathology and body mass index (BMI). They found that the rate of eating disorder diagnoses among the judged sport athletes was the highest, at 13 per cent, with the non-judged athletes and students each at 3 per cent.

There is, however, another reason why gymnasts and others in aesthetic sports strive to remain thin, and it is concerned with effective performance. Being lean is an advantage when it comes to performing the complex, 'high degree of difficulty' skilled moves that are required in international-level competition. Take, for example, Romanian gymnast Nadia Comaneci who, at the age of 14, won three gold, one silver and one bronze medal at the 1976 Summer Olympics in Montreal. Four years later at the Moscow games, she won two gold and two silver medals. Comaneci is remembered most for being the first gymnast to receive a perfect score of 10 for seven of her performances in Montreal. Later, she described the difficulty she had in performing complex skills as her body began to mature and she lost her thinness:

> I was an early developer, with hips and a chest that changed my centre of gravity, only a little, but enough to mean that moves that had once been effortless became torturous. For a gymnast, the arrival of puberty can be the end of an impossibly short career. The extra inches, or the pounds of fat can change you from a reliable, taut little performer into a gangly, clumsy lump who loses all sense of fluency and movement. For me, that meant the beginning of the end of my gym career – but for other young female gymnasts, training anywhere from America to China, puberty and weight-gain are held back to the detriment of their health.
> (*Observer*, 2005)

Research studies on gymnasts by Kerr *et al.* (2006) and Petrie (1993), and skaters by Monsma and Malina (2004) and Taylor and Ste-Marie (2001) are typical examples of a number of studies that have examined weight and disordered eating in samples of athletes in these specific sports. The results have been generally similar to those described earlier for aesthetic sport athletes as a group. They point to gymnasts and skaters having a desire to weigh less and be thin, being less satisfied with their bodies, using different and often uninformed types of dieting and weight control, and engaging in disordered eating behaviour to some extent, with the result that, in some athletes, it develops into a full-blown eating disorder.

While most research studies focus on currently active athletes, a more inclusive approach was adopted by Kerr *et al.* (2006). They used survey techniques (including open-ended questions) not only with current female gymnasts, but also with retired gymnasts, coaches, parents and judges. A number of interesting results were obtained, beyond those found in other studies. There were considerable discrepancies between the responses of the different respondent groups. For instance, current gymnasts reported fewer eating disorders and negative views of their experiences than were reported by the retired gymnasts. However, the most important findings concerned the gymnastic coaches, even though far fewer coaches (19 per cent) responded to the survey than any other group.

For example, none of the coaches who responded admitted using unhealthy weight control practices, but 82 per cent stated that other coaches used regular weighing, 43 per cent said others used public weighing, and 64 per cent said others kept private weight records. Also, 75 per cent of coaches said other coaches assessed body fat, but only one stated that he did so himself (Kerr *et al.*, 2006). As one of the respondent parents said:

> After learning that my daughter was underweight for her age, I told the coach the constant weighing had to stop. But the coaches want all control and the parents are to have none. I would not encourage my grandchildren or anyone else to go into this sport unless I saw a great change in coaching style.
>
> (Kerr *et al.*, 2006, p. 33)

In this study, 44 per cent of current gymnasts overheard coaches making negative comments about gymnasts' bodies, and those who were the target of disparaging comments about their bodies, or who received instructions to lose weight, were found to have significantly more disordered eating patterns than those who had not. Three per cent of current gymnasts and 20 per cent of retired gymnasts admitted to past or current eating disorders, and 73 per cent of retirees stated that they had suffered or were currently suffering from disordered eating behaviours. Lastly, some coaches discouraged their current athletes from completing the survey, and the authors speculated that it was likely that coaches who made use of unhealthy practices avoided completing the survey. The researchers wrote: 'In conclusion, it is clear from this study and others that disordered eating behaviours occur in gymnastics and are often endorsed, either implicitly or explicitly, by coaches and the sport context' (Kerr *et al.*, 2006, p. 40). This conclusion emphasizes the influential role that coaches can play in their interactions with young female gymnasts, giving their charges the perception that being thin and getting thinner will increase their performance scores.

Research studies on disordered eating have generally tended to group gymnasts under one label and examine them as a single entity. One UK study, however, actually compared female athletes in three different disciplines of gymnastics: artistic, rhythmic and sports acrobatics (Nordin *et al.*, 2003). For females, artistic gymnastics involves four activities: vaulting, short routines on the floor, asymmetric bars and balance beam. Rhythmic gymnastics has five activities, involving floor routines with ball, ribbon, hoop, clubs and rope. Sports acrobatics athletes take part in pairs or groups performing routines that include dance and tumbling moves as well as balances and tempo exercises. Fifty club-level athletes aged between 10 and 15 years, actively training and competing, took part in the study. Athletes completed the *perfectionism, drive for thinness, bulimia* and *body dissatisfaction* subscales from the EDI as well as providing researchers with other information about their participation in gymnastics. The results showed that, of the three, rhythmic gymnasts reported significantly higher *drive for thinness* scores and total eating disturbance scores than artistic gymnasts and sports acrobats. Also, perfectionism was found to be positively related to eating disturbance scores. Examining individual scores, the authors identified seven girls (14 per cent) who were at risk for developing eating disorders and, of these, four were rhythmic gymnasts and three were sports acrobats. The authors concluded that, considering their overall results, rhythmic gymnasts were the most at risk for developing eating disorders. Similar results were found in a previous study of twelve rhythmic gymnasts, where two were diagnosed as anorexic, two met the criteria for anorexia athletica and two others regularly fasted, vomited or used laxatives (Sundgot-Borgen, 1996).

With regard to the sports categorized in the aesthetic sport group, searches of the scientific research literature suggest that more research on eating disorders has been carried out on gymnasts than most of the other sports. From the studies reviewed here, it is clear that parents need to remain alert to the sometimes dubious weight control strategies of coaches and monitor the eating habits of their child athletes. Some coaches may set aside the ethical treatment of their charges in the pursuit of trying to produce winning athletes. This can have a detrimental effect on the health of the athletes and, if some do develop eating disorders, the effects can last for years. The threat to athletes' health is further underlined in the next section, which looks at weight-dependent sports.

Weight-dependent sports

In Sundgot-Borgen's (1993, 1994a, 1994b) research on female elite athletes, the weight-dependent category included athletes from judo, karate and wrestling, but boxers and athletes in some other sports, such as horse racing jockeys, could easily be added. The common element in these sports is that the athletes involved have to maintain their weight below a certain level in order to ensure their continued qualification for competition within particular weight classification divisions in their sports. This means that as well as keeping a continual check on their weight, some athletes engage in unhealthy practices, such as vomiting and the improper use of diuretics and laxatives. In boxing, for example, it is well known that boxers often have to undertake quite drastic weight reduction just before a fight to 'make their weight'. Athletes who persist with these unhealthy practices are putting themselves at risk for developing eating disorders. From the material presented below, and in support of Sundgot-Borgen's (1993, 1994a, 1994b) findings, it is apparent that a good number of those athletes participating in sports in this category have developed anorexia or bulimia, or a combination of both. For example, Lovett (1990) described the case of a 15-year-old male amateur boxer:

> David gave a history of a preoccupation with maintaining a low body weight from the age of about 14 years six months. His identified target weight (8 st 2 lb) lay just below the 25th centile for his age and height (Tanner and Whitehouse, 1959). He said he needed to stay at this weight to remain in the A.B.A. flyweight boxing division. His father took an active part in encouraging this, being involved in the weighing-in prior to each bout. David had dieted to achieve his present weight (8 st 4 lb). He only admitted to bingeing in our third session. His natural parents described David stealing food and bingeing on sweet foods, whilst his foster parents recounted how David kept his packed lunch to eat on his own in his room after a normal supper. David said that he tried to eat foods that made him feel full. He reported that self-induced vomiting was a common method amongst boxers of keeping their weight low, especially just before a fight. When the author first interviewed David, his vomiting took place after every meal, was secretive and was reported to be out of control. However, David's history showed that his vomiting behaviour was not always the same. In his family of origin he had regularly vomited in the kitchen sink and left the vomitus for his mother to find, and one family crisis was marked by his vomiting out of an upstairs window over the garage roof. In school David had used his vomiting like a party trick, a number of times vomiting in the playground in front of a group of girls in response to a 'dare'. David exercised regularly, spending a considerable amount of his time weight lifting.
>
> (Lovett, 1990, p. 80)

It is perhaps not surprising that David did satisfy the diagnostic criteria for bulimia, but following therapeutic work involving some psychotherapy and a behavioural programme, he made a speedy recovery from the condition. Part of this programme consisted of David giving up boxing and receiving three regular meals a day, after which he was not allowed to leave the room for an hour. This stopped him from visiting the toilet to induce vomiting. Six months after his first assessment, he was eating normally, had not vomited for three months, and weighed ten stone (i.e. 140 pounds) (Lovett, 1990).

In wrestling, quick weight loss is known as 'weight cutting' and it was thought to be responsible for the deaths of three US collegiate wrestlers in 1997. The three athletes, at universities in North Carolina, Wisconsin and Michigan, were attempting to lose weight by wearing rubber suits and exercising vigorously in hot environments, as part of a programme of rapid weight loss. Apparently, their coaches were present (Dick *et al.*, 2001; McKinney, 2005). They had each dropped their weights considerably over the previous two to three months and were trying to lose even more weight over a three- to twelve-hour period. One, who died of cardiac arrest, lost 19 pounds in four days and had hopes of losing another six pounds in order to wrestle at 190 pounds. These deaths were a shock to the NCAA wrestling community. Rule changes were quickly implemented in 1998 and a new wrestling weight management policy was drawn up (Dick *et al.*, 2001). Research has shown that these weight loss practices were not isolated cases. In a survey of 713 high school wrestlers, 45 per cent reported using weight cutting practices, with wrestlers on average losing 3.2 kilograms before competing, weight cycling 1.8 kilograms weekly, and fasting 20 hours prior to weigh-in. Restricting fluid intake, the use of rubber suits and vomiting were also found to be used by large numbers of high school wrestlers (Opplinger *et al.*, 1993). Research on 741 wrestlers, carried out in 1999 after the policy change, did suggest that weight loss behaviours have become less extreme, with 40 per cent of wrestlers found to be curbing their weight loss practices because of the new NCAA rules (Opplinger *et al.*, 2003).

It is perhaps hard to believe, but in spite of this trend to moderate weight loss practices in wrestling, Sansome and Sawyer (2005) reported a case of a five-year-old boy who was being pressured by his father to lose weight in order to wrestle in a lower weight class. The boy was a member of his local wrestling club, following in the footsteps of his 15-year-old brother, who had won a national wrestling award. His father, who had also been a wrestler, attended every competition and was actively involved in both their wrestling activities. The boy's coach overheard some of his comments and questions at the weigh-ins for the final competition of the season. The comments were about eating before being weighed, spending time in the sauna and not eating anything on that day or the day before. Alerted by these comments, the coach contacted the father and discussed the comments with him. The coach pointed out that there was a rule that stated that: 'at any time the use of sweat boxes, hot showers, whirlpools, rubber, vinyl and plastic-type suits; or other similar artificial heating devices . . . is prohibited and shall disqualify an individual from competition' (National Federation of State High Schools Associations, 2002). The coach later discovered that the major reason for the father pressurizing the son to lose weight was because he had lost to an opponent in a previous match, and by going down to a lower weight class, he could avoid a match with this particular opponent in the final competition of the season. This is an extreme instance of the influence a parent can have on the attitude and behaviour of a very young athlete, and the extremes to which parents are sometimes prepared to go to ensure their children's success in sport in contravention of both the rules of competition and the interests of their children's health.

Although other published research results demonstrating the existence of eating disorders in wrestlers are available (e.g. Opplinger *et al.*, 1993; Thiel *et al.*, 1993), some contradictory research results have been also been obtained. For example, in the Dale and Landers (1999) study, interviews with in-season wrestlers who scored above the EDI *drive for thinness* subscale 'at risk' cut-off point revealed that their concern with weight did not meet the diagnostic criteria for bulimia and were due solely to the demands of wrestling. However, even if wrestlers do not meet the criteria for eating disorders, the fact that many are engaging in weight cutting behaviour is a major cause for concern.

Horse racing jockeys are another group who are subject to very strict weight restrictions. In the world of the jockey, 'flipping' or 'heaving' is the term used for vomiting up what little they eat and, in the US, it is not uncommon for one of the toilets in the jockeys' room to be set aside for this purpose (Schmidt, 2004). Jockeys engage in vomiting, restrict what they eat and drink, and use the same rapid weight loss techniques as wrestlers. At least two deaths are thought to have been caused by these extreme measures. In 1991, an Australian jockey suffered a heart attack induced by using the race track's sauna, and in 2000, an American jockey died from heart arrhythmia because of low potassium levels caused by dieting (Schmidt, 2004).

When jockeys go on the scale to be weighed, they have to be wearing their riding gear and carrying their tack as well. In the US, the racing weight is usually in the range of 112–126 pounds, including the saddles and other gear, which usually weighs about seven pounds. In Britain, racing weights are three to four pounds heavier than in the US. As they mature, the majority of jockeys face a constant struggle to keep their weight down to the required levels and many develop health problems as a result. Some develop eating disorders such as bulimia (Fountaine, 2000; Hughes, 2006). For example, Herb McCauley, a former top jockey who rode more than 20,000 races, won more than 3,000 and made $70 million in winnings, suffered from bulimia for 20 years. He managed to recover when he retired from riding, but during his career he used a laxative called 'Ex-Lax' and a diuretic called 'Lasix' in addition to vomiting. He stated:

> 'I tried everything. I took so many slabs of Ex-Lax that to this day I can't eat a Hershey bar.' When commenting about Lasix, he said: 'That takes five to six pounds off, but it also takes all the fluids, electrolytes and minerals out of your body. All of a sudden your body cramps up and you're not the jockey you're supposed to be. You come down the stretch and think a hot poker is going through your hips.'
>
> (Fountaine, 2000, p. 2)

Steve Cauthen, another one of the most successful American jockeys, moved to England in 1979 and became a champion jockey there as well. Eventually, even the battle to meet the slightly higher weight requirements in England became too much and he retired early:

> That was the toughest thing about racing for me. I wasn't afraid of getting hurt. I loved the thrill, the competition, the glory and the glamour. But weight was the most negative side of my whole career.
>
> (Fountaine, 2000, p. 3)

Aaron Gryder, a leading US jockey, sticks to a strict diet of toast or fruit for breakfast, skips lunch and has a salad or a piece of chicken for dinner, but still has to drop two or three pounds on race days (Fountaine, 2000). Gryder stated:

> If you walked into a health food store and looked at a chart, it would say someone my height [5 feet 6 inches] and [age] 29 should weigh 140 pounds – not 112. The sauna might be nice for 15 minutes, but it's not a healthy place to be five times a week, all day.
>
> (Fountaine, 2000, p. 1)

Research studies carried out in three different countries (England, New Zealand and Australia) have produced results that tend to confirm the anecdotal statements from individual jockeys such as McCauley, Cauthen and Gryder. All three studies (King and Mezey, 1987; Leydon and Wall, 2002; Moore *et al.*, 2002) confirm the widespread use of rapid weight loss techniques by jockeys to reduce their weight, especially just prior to racing. These techniques include skipping meals on a regular basis and, before racing, restricting food and fluid intake, using saunas and hot baths, laxatives, diuretics and appetite suppressants. For example, the English study (King and Mezey, 1987) found that jockeys' weights were well below matched population mean weights and found an average EAT measure score that was significantly higher than that reported for males in other studies. Follow-up psychiatric interviews with ten jockeys revealed that bingeing was common, but vomiting was relatively unusual among this small sample of English jockeys. Nevertheless, it appears that, like the wrestlers and boxers discussed above, jockeys are almost forced to engage in mandatory unhealthy eating practices in order to survive in the sport. It is hardly surprising that some develop eating disorders in an environment where vomiting and other methods of losing weight rapidly are so commonplace that they are unremarkable to those in racing.

Endurance sports

Long distance running, swimming, cycling, biathlon, cross-country skiing, orienteering, race walking, rowing, speed skating over long distances, triathlon and possibly weight training would qualify for inclusion in this category. Focusing on one of these sports, long distance running, anecdotal reports from other elite runners support Sundgot-Borgen's (1993, 1994a, 1994b) research findings. Alison Outram, a former international British runner who competed in the World Junior Cross-Country championships in 1996 after years of hard training, was an athlete who suffered from an eating disorder during her athletic career. In 1998, at the age of 21, her body was so weak that she sometimes had difficulty walking and at times had to use a wheelchair (Downes, 1998):

I have an addictive personality, like many people with eating disorders, and I became obsessional about training. I ran more, ate less. For a while my results improved and my self-esteem grew while my self-hate began to disintegrate slightly . . . I kept running internationally for as long as I could, until I saw a specialist who told me that I might only have one week to live. I reached a stage where if I was running well, nothing else mattered. Consequently I neglected my well-being.

(Downes, 1998, p. 54)

It seems that Outram was not an isolated case. Thirty-five teenage girls had represented Britain at the Junior World Cross-Country Championships in the six years prior to 1998, but only four moved on to compete in senior events. When British Athletics checked up, they found that 17 of the 35 runners had experienced some form of eating disorder (Downes, 1998). Liz McColgan, the British 10,000-metre runner who ran at the 1988 Seoul Olympics, was thought to have a good chance of winning the gold medal. However, an eating disorder prevented her from achieving her goal and she ended up with a silver medal:

I had never been obsessed with my weight, but I was always obsessed with running faster. During the run-up to the Seoul games, my coach told me I could lose a few pounds. It started a snowball effect. In my mind the thinner I became, the faster I could run . . . I ran for my life, but because I was so weak and under-nourished I struggled at the end. I didn't have the energy to sprint for gold.

(Downes, 1998, p. 55)

Research carried out by Yates *et al.* (1983) and Yates (1991) drew attention to and confirmed the link between exercise (more specifically, running) and eating disorders. Their research involved in-depth interviews with some 150 male and female runners and, based on these interviews, a number of illustrative cases of 'obligatory' runners were presented in Yates (1991). One typical case, the case of Patty that was included in Chapter 1, could equally well have been placed in this current chapter. Patty was an eight-mile a day runner who ran to counterbalance the food she ate the day before and, like the wrestlers and jockeys described above, also used laxatives or enemas to keep her weight down.

Other research, using different methods, has concentrated specifically on elite distance runners. By way of illustration, a South African study used the EAT and EDI measures with a group of 115 female marathon runners, elite ultra-marathon runners, cross-country runners and a control group of non-runners (Weight and Noakes, 1987). They found a low incidence of anorexia in the overall group, but 18 runners were found to have abnormal eating attitudes symptomatic of anorexia and one had been treated for anorexia. Five more of these 18 athletes (including three elite marathon runners and a highly ranked track athlete) had low body mass and amenorrhea. A second study provided stronger evidence. The researchers examined 181 athletes from the top of the respective rankings for UK middle and long distance races in 1996–97 and included track, road, cross-country and fell/mountain running athletes (Hulley and Hill, 2001). The athletes completed the Eating Disorder Examination Questionnaire (EDE-Q; Fairburn and Beglin, 1994) and answered questions on demographics, athletic training, diet and health. Seven athletes were found to be anorexic, two had bulimia and twenty had eating disorders not otherwise specified (EDNOS). In addition, six other athletes had previously received treatment for eating disorders. The findings of these two questionnaire studies (Hulley and Hill, 2001; Weight and Noakes, 1987) are consistent with the findings from Yates' (1991) interview-based case studies and the anecdotal comments of the elite runners, Outram and McColgan. It appears that some athletes in endurance sports, like their peers in aesthetic and weight dependent sports, are susceptible to developing eating disorders.

Additional issues

Body dissatisfaction

Body dissatisfaction is one of the subscales on the EDI and it is well known that in general, one of the characteristics of anorexics is that their image of their own bodies becomes distorted and, although they are very thin, they often perceive their bodies as being much fatter than they actually are. This pattern holds up well with, for example, track, cross-country, gymnastics and skating athletes with eating problems who are often dissatisfied with their builds because they are not small or thin enough. However, with weight trainers, body builders (e.g. Blouin and Goldfield, 1995) and athletes in some other sports (e.g. American football players; Johnson *et al.*, 1999), the feelings of body dissatisfaction come from not being big enough. While some people have a drive for thinness, others have a drive for muscularity (Ricciardelli and McCabe, 2004).

There have been reported cases of 'obligatory' weight lifters (individuals who spend numerous hours per week working out in gyms, lifting weights and using muscle building machines) who have eating disorders (e.g. Pasman and Thompson, 1988). Seheult (1995), describing her assessment of the psychological difficulties experienced by a client who was a 'body-building addict', outlined his particular approach to diet:

> In general this diet consisted of a very limited range of food – pasta, rice and tuna fish. Talking to Mr E it seemed that the imposition of this very stringent dieting had created for him a somewhat distorted attitude toward food which at certain times he had come only to see as 'fuel' for the moulding of his body into the desired form. Although

describing himself as 'fed up' with eating pasta, tuna and rice, he did not seem to have any real idea of what he would prefer to eat. He did his own cooking . . . As far as he saw it, the weight and strength training developed muscle bulk and the restricted high protein diet reduced fat levels thus providing the much desired muscle definition for which competitive body-builders all strive.

(Seheult, 1995, pp. 41–2)

Weight trainers' and bodybuilders' behaviour, with its extreme focus on diet, body fat and excessive exercise, resembles anorexic behaviour to some degree. This is perhaps not surprising, as it has been shown that the personality characteristics of anorexic females and male body builders are very similar. Both groups were found to be significantly more obsessional, perfectionist, anhedonic and pathologically narcissistic than the general population (Davis and Scott-Robinson, 2000). The one interesting exception was that the anorexics had negative perceptions while the body builders had very positive perceptions of self-worth. There is, of course, another major difference, and that is that the anorexic's drive for thinness is replaced by the body builder's drive to develop lean muscle mass by losing fat and developing muscle. This has been termed 'reverse anorexia' (Pope *et al.*, 1993) and, in some cases where an individual develops a disorder where he or she becomes obsessed by the perception that they are not muscular enough, as 'muscle dysmorphia' (e.g. Hardy, 1982; Ricciardelli and McCabe, 2004). Therefore, distortion of body image and body dissatisfaction can work in different ways for athletes in different sports. However, it should be noted that research has shown that the female drive for thinness and the male drive for muscularity are characterized by similar psychological profiles, especially with regard to neuroticism and perfectionism (Davis *et al.*, 2005).

Eating disorders and high-level performance

There is some debate about the ability of elite athletes with eating disorders to maintain high-level performance. Thompson and Sherman (1993) have argued that some athletes are still able to perform at high levels, in spite of the severe psychological and physiological problems that accompany anorexia. However, Sundgot-Borgen (1994a) pointed out that although it is assumed that some of the risk factors for the development of eating disorders, such as intense pressure to be lean, increased training volume and perfectionism, are likely to be greater in elite athletes, they would have difficulty in performing at that level for any length of time with a severe eating disorder, as performance would deteriorate. This was certainly true in the case of retired jockey Herb McCauley and the extreme case of US gymnast Christy Henrich, described earlier. Intuitively, it makes sense that the effects of eating disorders would eventually catch up with an athlete and affect performance detrimentally (Beals, 2004). Further, it is possible that athletes who have failed to stay at the elite level are more likely to have problems associated with eating disorders than those who are able to maintain their performance at that level (Sundgot-Borgen, 1994a). Additional research with elite, sub-elite and 'failing' elite athletes might help to clarify these issues.

Female athlete triad syndrome

The so-called 'female athlete triad' syndrome is a cause for concern among the sport medicine fraternity, to the extent that the American College of Sports Medicine (ACSM) has published a position statement on the female athlete triad (Otis *et al.*, 1997). The triad is comprised of three interrelated medical disorders (disordered eating, amenorrhea and osteoporosis) often found in female athletes. The position statement underlines the fact that 'adolescents and women training in sports in which low body weight is emphasized for athletic activity or appearance are at greatest risk' (Otis *et al.*, 1997, p. i). Although no sport is thought to be immune, the types of sports identified by Otis *et al.* (1997) as having athletes most at risk for developing the female athlete triad are the same ones recognized in this chapter for eating disorders, namely those included within the aesthetic, weight-dependent and endurance sports categories. It is also worth noting that the ACSM position statement goes on to recommend that athletes found to have one component of the triad should be screened for the other two components.

Distinct symptomatology for athletes

A query that sometimes crops up in discussion among sport psychologists is whether athletes with eating disorders actually share the same psychopathological characteristics as ordinary people who have eating disorder conditions. In partial answer to this question, the results of a study in which eating-disordered female patients who had been involved in high-level competitive athletics were compared with females with eating disorders who were non-athletes identified no significant statistical differences between the two groups on any eating-related symptoms or measures of psychopathology. In other words, the two groups not only shared symptoms such as dieting and fear of weight gain, but also had similar psychopathological characteristics. Davis and Strachan (2001) concluded that the psychological profile of female athletes who develop an eating disorder is no different from other females with eating disorders.

Closing comments

In Chapter 1, several sports events were mentioned as being examples of the types of sports where individuals with exercise dependence were likely to be found. These events included the Western States' 100-mile Endurance Run, the Run across America 2004 'race', fell racing in the Lake District in England and the Hawaii Ironman triathlon event. In Chapter 3, evidence was presented to show how the addiction process might work through the positive changes in hedonic tone that can accompany participation in exercise activities (Brown, 1997, 2001). In Chapter 4, it was argued that eating disorders were forms of addictions or dependencies similar to gambling or drinking alcohol. In the present chapter, taking the discussion a step further, other evidence has been collated to show that athletes in certain sports are at risk for developing eating disorders, and it seems that many of the factors associated with eating disorders in general are exacerbated in athletes. This progression has been followed in an attempt to develop a well-reasoned argument to show that not only do athletes run the risk of developing exercise dependence, but some, at least, are also at risk for developing eating disorders, or a combination of both. In the following chapter, a further piece of the exercise dependence puzzle is put in place when the underlying personality characteristics of primary and secondary exercise dependent athletes are examined.

References

American Psychiatric Association (APA) (1994) *Diagnostic and statistical manual of mental disorders* (4th edition), Washington DC: American Psychiatric Association.

Beals, K. A. (2004) *Disordered eating among athletes*, Champaign IL: Human Kinetics.

Blouin, A. G. and Goldfield, G. S. (1995) 'Body image and steroid use in male bodybuilders', *International Journal of Eating Disorders*, 18, 159–65.

Brown, R. I. F. (1997) 'A theoretical model of behavioural addictions – Applied to offending', in J. E. Hodge, M. McMurran and C. R. Hollin (eds) *Addicted to crime?*, New York: Wiley, 13–65.

Brown, R. I. F. (2001) 'Addictions', in M. J. Apter (ed.) *Motivational styles in everyday life: A guide to reversal theory*, Washington DC: American Psychological Association, 155–65.

Dale, K. S. and Landers, D. M. (1999) 'Weight control in wrestling: eating disorders or disordered eating?', *Medicine and Science in Sports and Exercise*, 31, 1382–9.

Davis, C. and Scott-Robinson, L. (2000) 'A psychological comparison of females with anorexia nervosa and competitive male body builders: Body shape ideals in the extreme', *Eating Behaviors*, 1, 33–46.

Davis, C. and Strachan, S. (2001) 'Elite female athletes with eating disorders: A study of psychopathological characteristics', *Journal of Sport & Exercise Psychology*, 23, 245–53.

Davis, C., Karvinen, K. and McCreary, D. R. (2005) 'Personality correlates of a drive for muscularity in young men', *Personality and Individual Differences*, 39, 349–59.

DiBartolo, P. M. and Shaffer, C. (2002) 'A comparison of female college athletes and nonathletes: Eating disorder symptomology and psychological well-being', *Journal of Sport and Exercise Psychology*, 24, 33–41.

Dick, R.W., Opplinger, R. A., Scott, J. R. and Utter, A. C. (2001) *Wrestling with weight loss: The NCAA wrestling weight management policy*. Online. Available www. ncaa.org/library/sports_sciences.

Downes, S. (1998) 'Running on empty', *Running Times*, October, 53–6.

Fairburn, C. and Beglin, S. J. (1994) 'The assessment of eating disorders: Interview or self-report questionnaire?', *International Journal of Eating Disorders*, 16, 363–70.

Fountaine, E. (2000) 'Stakes are high for overweight jockeys', *New York Thoroughbred Horsemens Association Newsletter*, June. Online. Available www.nytha.com.

Fulkerson, J. A., Keel, P. K., Leon, G. and Dorr, T. (1999) 'Eating-disordered behaviors and personality characteristics of high school athletes and nonathletes', *International Journal of Eating Disorders*, 26, 73–9.

Garner, D. M. (1991) *Eating Disorder Inventory-2*, Odessa FL: Psychological Assessment Resources.

Garner, D. M. and Olmsted, M. P. (1984) *Eating Disorder Inventory manual*, Odessa FL: Psychological Assessment Resources.

Garner, D. M., Olmsted, M. P., Bohr, Y. and Garfinkel, P. E. (1982) 'The Eating Attitudes Test: Psychometric features and clinical correlates', *Psychological Medicine*, 12, 871–8.

Garner, D. M., Olmsted, M. P. and Polivy, J. (1983) 'Development and validation of a multi-dimensional Eating Disorder Inventory for anorexia nervosa and bulimia', *International Journal of Eating Disorders*, 2, 15–34.

Grogan. S. (1999) *Body image: Understanding body dissatisfaction in men, women and children*, New York: Routledge.

Haase, A. M., Prapavessis, H. and Owens, R. Glynn (2002) 'Perfectionism, social physique anxiety and disordered eating: a comparison of male and female athletes', *Psychology of Sport and Exercise*, 3, 209–22.

Hardy, G. E. (1982) 'Body image disturbance in dysmorphophobia', *British Journal of Psychiatry*, 141, 181–5.

Hausenblas, H. A. and Carron, A. V. (1999) 'Eating disorder indices and athletes: An integration', *Journal of Sport and Exercise Psychology*, 21, 230–58.

Hughes, R. (2006) 'Are weight limits putting the health of jockeys at risk?', *The Guardian*, 3 May. Online. Available http://sport.guardian.co.uk.

Hulley, A. J. and Hill, A. J. (2001) 'Eating disorders and health in elite woman distance runners', *International Journal of Eating Disorders*, 30, 312–17.

Japan Times (1994) '"Monster" inside Henrich never let go', 29 September, 22.

Johnson, C. (1985) 'Initial consultation for patients with bulimia and anorexia nervosa', in D. M. Garner and P. E. Garfinkel (eds) *Handbook of psychotherapy of anorexia nervosa and bulimia*, New York: Guilford Press, 19–54.

Johnson, C., Powers, P. S. and Dick, R. (1999) 'Athletes and eating disorders: The National Collegiate Athletic Association study', *International Journal of Eating Disorders*, 26, 179–88.

Kerr, G., Berman, E. and De Souza, M. J. (2006) 'Disordered eating in women's gymnastics: Perspectives of athletes, coaches, parents, and judges', *Journal of Applied Sport Psychology*, 18, 28–43.

King, M. B. and Mezey, G. (1987) 'Eating behaviour of male racing jockeys', *Psychological Medicine*, 17, 249–53.

Langley, J. (2006) *Boys get anorexia too: Coping with male eating disorders in the family*, London: Paul Chapman.

Leydon, M. A. and Wall, C. (2002) New Zealand jockeys' dietary habits and their potential impact on health, *International Journal of Sport Nutrition and Exercise Metabolism*, 12, 220–37.

Lovett, J. W. T. (1990) 'Bulimia nervosa in an adolescent boy boxer', *Journal of Adolescence*, 13, 79–83.

McKinney, E. (2005) 'Weighing in on wrestling'. Online. Available www.sun-herald.com/Newsarchive.

Manore, M. and Thompson, J. (2000) *Sport nutrition for health and performance*, Champaign IL: Human Kinetics.

Monsma, E. V. and Malina, R. M. (2004) 'Correlates of eating disorders risk among female figure skates: A profile of adolescent competitors', *Psychology of Sport and Exercise*, 5, 447–60.

Moore, J. M., Timperio, A. F., Crawford, D. A., Burns, C. M. and Cameron-Smith, D. (2002) 'Weight management and weight loss strategies of professional jockeys', *International Journal of Sport Nutrition and Exercise Metabolism*, 12, 1–13.

National Federation of State High Schools Associations, (2002) *Wrestling 2002–2003 rules book*, Indianapolis IN: National Federation of State High Schools Associations.

Nordin, S. M., Harris, G. and Cumming, J. (2003) 'Disturbed eating in young competitive gymnasts: Differences between three gymnastics disciplines', *European Journal of Sport Science*, 3, 1–14.

Observer (2005) 'Growing pains', 4 December. Online. Available http://observer.guardian.co.uk.

Opplinger, R. A., Landry, G. L., Foster, S. W. and Lambrecht, A. C. (1993) 'Bulimic behaviours among interscholastic wrestlers: A statewide survey', *Pediatrics*, 91, 826–31.

Opplinger, R. A., Steen, S. A. and Scott, J. R. (2003) 'Weight loss practices of college wrestlers', *International Journal of Sport Nutrition and Exercise Metabolism*, 13, 29–46.

Otis, C. L., Drinkwater, B., Johnson, M., Loucks, A. and Wilmore, J. (1997) 'ACSM position stand: The female athlete triad', *Medicine in Science and Sports and Exercise*, 29, i-ix.

Pasman, L. and Thompson, J. K. (1988) 'Body and eating disturbance in obligatory runners, obligatory weightlifters, and sedentary individuals', *International Journal of Eating Disorders*, 7, 759–69.

Petrie, T. (1993) 'Disordered eating in female collegiate gymnasts: Prevalence and personality/attitudinal correlates', *Journal of Sport and Exercise Psychology*, 15, 424–36.

Petrie, T. A. and Rogers, R. (2001) 'Extending the discussion of eating disorders to include men and athletes', *The Counseling Psychologist*, 5, 743–53.

Picard, C. L. (1999) 'The level of competition as a factor for the development of eating disorders in female collegiate athletes', *Journal of Youth and Adolescence*, 28, 583–94.

Pope, H. G., Katz, D. L. and Hudson, J. I. (1993) 'Anorexia nervosa and "reverse anorexia" among 108 male bodybuilders', *Comprehensive Psychiatry*, 34, 406–9.

Ricciardelli, L. A. and McCabe, M. P. (2004) 'A biopsychosocial model of disordered eating and the pursuit of muscularity in adolescent boys', *Psychological Bulletin*, 130, 179–205.

Ryan, J. (1995) *Little girls in pretty boxes: The making and breaking of elite gymnasts and figure skaters*, New York: Doubleday.

Ryan, J. (1996) *Little girls in pretty boxes: The making and breaking of elite gymnasts and figure skaters*, London: The Women's Press.

Sansome, R. A. and Sawyer, R. (2005) 'Weightloss pressure on a 5 year old wrestler', *British Journal of Sports Medicine*, 39, e2. Online case reports. Available http://bjsm.bmjjournals.com.

Schmidt, N. (2004) 'Horse racing's dirty little secret', *The Cincinnati Enquirer*, 25 April. Online. Available www.enquirer.com.

Seheult, C. (1995) 'Hooked on the "Buzz": History of a body-building addict', in J. Annett, B. Cripps and H. Steinberg (eds) *Exercise addiction: Motivation for participation in sport and exercise*, Leicester: The British Psychological Society, 41–2.

Smolak, L., Murnen, S. K. and Ruble, A. E. (2000) 'Female athletes and eating problems: a meta-analysis', *International Journal of Eating Disorders*, 27, 371–80.

Sundgot-Borgen, J. (1993) 'Prevalence of eating disorders in female elite athletes', *International Journal of Sport Nutrition*, 3, 29–40.

Sundgot-Borgen, J. (1994a) 'Eating disorders in female athletes', *Sports Medicine*, 17, 176–88.

Sundgot-Borgen, J. (1994b) 'Risk and trigger factors for the development of eating disorders in female elite athletes', *Medicine and Science in Sports and Exercise*, 26, 414–19.

Sundgot-Borgen, J. (1996) 'Eating disorders, energy intake, training volume, and menstrual function in high-level modern rhythmic gymnasts', *International Journal of Sport Nutrition*, 6, 100–9.

Sundgot-Borgen, J., Torstveit, G. and Klungland, M. (2004) 'Prevalence of eating disorders in elite athletes is higher than in the general population', *Clinical Journal of Sport Medicine*, 14, 25–32.

Tanner, J. M. and Whitehouse, R. H. (1959) *Height and weight standard charts*, Middlesex: Printwell Press.

Taube D. E. and Blinde, E. M. (1992) 'Eating disorders among adolescent female athletes: Influence of athletic participation and sport team membership', *Adolescence*, 27, 833–48.

Taylor, G. M. and Ste-Marie, D. M. (2001) 'Eating disorders symptoms in Canadian pair and dance figure skaters', *International Journal of Sport Psychology*, 32, 21–8.

Thiel, A., Gottfried, H. and Heese, F. W. (1993) 'Subclinical eating disorders in male athletes. A study of the low weight category in rowers and wrestlers', *Acta Psychiatrica Scandinavica*, 88, 259–65.

Thompson, R. A. and Sherman, R. T. (1993) *Helping athletes with eating disorders*, Champaign IL: Human Kinetics.

Weight, L. M. and Noakes, T. D. (1987) 'Is running an analog of anorexia? A survey of the incidence in female distance runners', *Medicine and Science in Sports and Exercise*, 19, 213–17.

Yates, A. (1991) *Compulsive exercise and the eating disorders*, New York: Brunner Mazel.

Yates, A., Leehey, K. and Shisslak, C. M. (1983) 'Running: An analogue of anorexia?', *The New England Journal of Medicine*, 308, 251–5.

Zucker, N. L., Womble, L. G., Williamson, D. A. and Perrin, L. A. (1999) 'Protective factors for eating disorders in female college athletes', *Eating Disorders: The Journal of Treatment and Prevention*, 7, 207–18.

6 Hooked on exercise

Personality and motivation in primary and secondary exercise dependence

Comprehensive research work on exercise dependent people has taken place in at least three centres widely dispersed across the globe. One group, based at the University of Florida in the US, involved Hausenblas, Symons Downs and colleagues; a second, based at Birmingham University in England, involved Cockerill, Bamber and colleagues; and a third, at The University of Hong Kong, involved Blaydon, Lindner and Kerr. These three groups have produced a number of scientific publications over the last ten years.

The Florida group's work was mostly concerned with providing a comprehensive review of the exercise dependence literature (Hausenblas and Symons Downs, 2002a) and developing a new scale for measuring exercise dependence (Hausenblas and Symons Downs, 2002b), but one study examined the relationship between exercise dependence and personality (Hausenblas and Giacobbi, 2004).

The Birmingham-based work involved a review of the existing literature on exercise dependence (Cockerill and Riddington, 1996), as well as studies of physically active sports, dance or exercise participants. These studies used quantitative (Bamber et al., 2000a) and qualitative (Bamber et al., 2000b) methods, and screened participants for eating disorders. A fourth publication attempted to formulate diagnostic criteria for exercise dependence (Bamber et al., 2003). In the quantitative study, participants were divided into four different groups: exercise dependent; exercise dependent with an eating disorder; eating disordered; and controls (with neither exercise dependence nor eating disorders). They were compared on a number of variables, including personality (Bamber et al., 2000a). The Hong Kong research attempted to advance the previous work undertaken in Birmingham by repeating the general methodology of the quantitative Birmingham study (Bamber et al., 2000a), using reversal theory-based personality measures and more stringent exercise dependence criteria. One of two studies focused on an amateur sport sample (Blaydon et al., 2004) and the other on a specific sport, triathlon (Blaydon and Lindner, 2002; Blaydon et al., 2002). Qualitative data was also collected from primary and secondary exercise dependent exercisers, eating disordered exercisers and exercisers with no dependence (Blaydon, 2001).

In this chapter, the quantitative research carried out by these three research groups will be examined in more detail. While all the information accrued from these studies is potentially important, of particular interest are the findings that were obtained about the personality of exercise dependent individuals. They are of special interest because Brown (1997), in his Hedonic Management Model of Addictions, argued that some individuals are more vulnerable to addictions than others. He also argued that a person's 'hedonic gap' (the discrepancy between the level of negative feeling states (e.g. frustration, pain) a person can tolerate and the level they experience; see Chapter 2) plays an important role in individual vulnerability. In general, the wider a person's hedonic gap may be, the greater their vulnerability to addictions. Brown (1997) also described seven factors that he thought could contribute to the vulnerability of an individual; one of these was the role that individual differences in personality and temperament might play.

Exercise dependence and personality

The Florida study

This study, carried out by Hausenblas and Giacobbi (2004), administered a number of questionnaires to 390 US male and female undergraduate and postgraduate university students. These included the Exercise Dependence Scale (EDS; a 21-item scale derived from DSM-IV criteria for substance abuse, Hausenblas and Symons Downs, 2002b) and the *drive for thinness* subscale from the Eating Disorder Inventory-2 (EDI-2; Garner, 1991) to assess exercise dependence symptoms. The NEO Five Factor Inventory (NEO-FFI; Costa and McCrae, 1992a), measuring *neuroticism, extraversion, openness, agreeableness* and *conscientiousness*, was used to assess personality, and the Leisure-Time Exercise Questionnaire (LTEQ; Godin and Shephard, 1985) was used to measure the frequency of strenuous, moderate and mild leisure-time weekly exercise. Seventeen females who scored above 14 on the *drive for thinness* subscale (Garner, 1991) were excluded from further analysis by the authors in order to avoid the potential confounding effects of including participants with secondary exercise dependence. The data from the remaining 373 participants was analysed using correlation and hierarchical regression analysis procedures.

As far as personality was concerned, the results showed that NEO-FFI *extraversion* and *neuroticism* were found to be positively correlated, and *agreeableness* negatively correlated, with exercise dependence. Extraverted people tend to active, social, outgoing and spontaneous, and introverted people are quiet, passive, unsociable and inhibited. People scoring high on the *neuroticism* subscale tend to be anxious, rigid, worried, vulnerable and insecure as opposed to people who score low on this dimension, who tend to be more stable, calm, even-tempered and secure. High scores on the *agreeableness* subscale indicate people who tend to be good-natured, soft-hearted and selfless, whereas low scores indicate people who tend to be irritable, ruthless and selfish. Further analysis showed that these three subscales were significant predictors of primary exercise dependence symptoms.

In trying to explain these results, Hausenblas and Giacobbi (2004) argued that individuals scoring high on neuroticism are often irrational and have trouble coping with stress. These people may tend to be worried about their health or appearance and use exercise as a maladaptive coping strategy. They also argued that, as extraverted people are generally energetic, active and tend to like excitement and as exercise activities require these charac-teristics, it is not surprising that exercise dependent people report high scores on the extraversion scale. However, this argument is weak because it is well established in the exercise and sports psychology literature (e.g. Kerr, 1997) that different personality types prefer and perform different types of activities. Therefore, the argument would apply only to certain types of exercise and sport activities (e.g. explosive activities such as baseball and cricket) and not to others (e.g. endurance activities such as marathon running). The authors further suggested that disagreeable people become excessive exercisers to satisfy their competitive nature or, alternatively, that they might have exaggerated the truth in their EDS responses. The former suggestion is unjustifiable, and if the latter suggestion about exaggerated EDS responses is correct, this would also invalidate their other findings.

In addition, the authors themselves pointed to a number of shortcomings associated with their study. First, they questioned the accuracy of indirect measurement of exercise activity through the use of a questionnaire and recommended that objective measures of exercise be used by researchers. Second, they pointed out that the generalizability of the findings was limited because the study sample consisted of university students. Third, they indi-cated that causality cannot be established because of the nature of correla-tional studies and, fourth, that the short version (NEO-FFI) of the personality scale may be less reliable and valid than the full version (NEO-PI-R; Costa and McCrae, 1992a, 1992b). Consequently, there are a number of reasons why the results of this study are open to question.

The Birmingham study

The Birmingham researchers were interested in examining differences, in-cluding differences in personality, between primary (exercise dependence only) and secondary (exercise dependence and an eating disorder) exercise dependent individuals. A total of 194 young women comprised the sample in the study undertaken by Bamber *et al.* (2000a). The women came from a wide variety of exercise contexts (university aerobics dance classes; university and community sports centres; university cross-country and athletics clubs; local running clubs; readers of *Athletics Weekly* magazine; the *Runners World* magazine buddy scheme; and athletes from the UK Athletics Organization) and eating disorder groups (members of the Eating Disorders Association in the UK; patients with eating disorders from a private eating disorders clinic; and students with eating disorders from university counselling services).

Respondents completed a battery of questionnaires that included measures of exercise dependence (Exercise Dependence Questionnaire (EDQ); Ogden *et al.*, 1997), eating disorders (Eating Disorder Examination Questionnaire (EDE-Q); Fairburn and Beglin, 1994), psychological morbidity (General Health Questionnaire (GHQ-28); Goldberg and Williams, 1988), personality (Eysenck Personality Questionnaire-Revised, (EPQ-R); Eysenck and Eysenck, 1991), self-esteem (Rosenberg Self-Esteem Scale (RSES); Rosenberg, 1965), beliefs about exercise (Exercise Belief Questionnaire (EBQ); Loumidis and Wells, 1998), and attitudes to body shape (Body Shape Questionnaire (BSQ); Paa and Larson, 1998), as well as self-reports about weight dissatisfaction, menstrual functioning and physical activity levels. The EPQ-R, the question-naire measuring personality, has three main subscales; *extraversion-introversion* and *neuroticism-stability* are similar to the NEO-FFI factors of the same name, and high scores on the *psychoticism* subscale indicate a tendency to be solitary, troublesome and insensitive towards other people. In addition to a 'Lie scale' (designed to assess socially desirable responses), the other subscales measure *addictiveness* (tendency to become addicted), *venturesomeness* (sensation-seeking), *impulsiveness* (saying and doing things without thinking), and *empathy* (recognizing and sharing another person's emotions).

The EDQ (with a cut-off point of 116) and the EDE-Q were used in a methodology first suggested by Veale (1995) to classify respondents into primary exercise dependent (high EDQ-low EDE-Q), secondary exercise dependent (high EDQ-high EDE-Q), eating disordered (low EDQ-high EDE-Q) and control (low EDQ-low EDE-Q) groups. Chi-square procedures were used for analysing nominal data, and group comparisons on the variables described above were completed using Analysis of Variance (ANOVA) techniques with post hoc comparisons where appropriate.

The authors' interpretation of the results of the Birmingham study needs to be examined in some detail here. Although the authors concluded that 'the primary exercise dependence group was largely indistinguishable from the controls', and 'the secondary exercise dependence group … differed little from the eating disorder group' (Bamber *et al.*, 2002a, p. 125) and that the results 'argue against the notion that primary exercise dependence is a pathology' (p. 130), these conclusions did not seem to correspond with the findings reported in the published paper. Careful re-examination of their reported results indicates that, in reality, there were quite a number of important significant differences among all four groups. The primary exercise dependence group scored significantly higher than the control group on the *anxiety/insomnia* subscale of the GHQ-28, had more than double the controls' percentage of *amenorrhoea* cases, significantly higher concern about *body shape* (BSQ) than controls (but significantly less concern than the secondary exercise dependent and eating disordered groups), scored higher on the EPQ-R *neuroticism*, *addictiveness*, and *impulsiveness* subscales and on the EBQ total score (more maladaptive beliefs) and its *social desirability*, *physical appearance* and *mental/emotional functioning* subscales, and had a higher *physical activity level* score than the control group (see Table 6.1).

The secondary exercise dependence group differed from the eating disordered group in the following six variables: higher GHQ-28 *severe depression* subscale score, nearly double the incidence of *amenorrhoea*, higher on the EPQ-R *venturesomeness* subscale, higher on EBQ total score and its *social desirability* subscale, and had a higher *physical activity level* score (see Table 6.1).

In fact, the data as published indicated additional significant differences among the four groups, with the primary group scoring lower than the secondary group on most GHQ-28 variables, higher on RSES *self-esteem*, lower on *weight dissatisfaction*, lower on EBQ total score, *social desirability*, *physical appearance* and *mental/emotional functioning* subscales, lower on EPQ-R *neuroticism*, *addictiveness* and *impulsiveness* subscales, but higher on EPQ-R *extraversion* and *venturesomeness*. The secondary exercise dependence group differed significantly from the control group in most measures. The fewest differences were reported between the primary exercise dependence and the eating disordered groups. The primary exercise dependent group differed from the eating disordered group only in *self-esteem* (higher), *amenorrhoea* cases (higher), *body shape concern* (lower) and *physical activity levels* (higher).

A more accurate summary of Bamber *et al.*'s (2000a) findings is that there were substantial differences in psychological characteristics between the three groups with exercise and/or eating problems and the control group. In the

Table 6.1 Significant results for the primary exercise dependence group versus (1) the control group and (2) the secondary exercise dependence group in the Bamber *et al.* (2000a) study

Variables	
GHQ-28 anxiety/insomnia	Primary > Control
GHQ-28 subscales	Primary < Secondary on 3 out of 4
% amenorrhoea	Primary more than double Control
RSES self-esteem	Primary > Secondary
BSQ body shape concern	Primary < Control
weight dissatisfaction	Primary < Secondary
EPQ-R extraversion	Primary > Secondary
EPQ-R neuroticism	Primary > Control – Primary < Secondary
EPQ-R addictiveness	Primary > Control – Primary < Secondary
EPQ-R impulsiveness	Primary > Control – Primary < Secondary
EPQ-R venturesomeness	Primary > Secondary
EBQ total score	Primary > Control – Primary < Secondary
EBQ social desirability	Primary > Control – Primary < Secondary
EBQ physical appearance	Primary > Control – Primary < Secondary
EBQ mental/emotional function	Primary > Control – Primary < Secondary

light of these significant differences, it is hard to understand how the authors arrived at their conclusions. Primary exercise dependent females could be clearly distinguished from both controls and secondary exercise dependent females on a number of important variables and thus these results actually do support the recognition of primary exercise dependence as a separate pathological condition.

The study by Bamber *et al.* (2000a) provided some important data on the personality dimensions of primary and secondary exercise dependent individuals from the EPQ-R scale (see Table 6.1). Recapping briefly, controls differed significantly from the other three groups on *neuroticism* (lower), *addictiveness* (lower) and *impulsiveness* (lower). With regard to *extraversion*, controls were only significantly higher than the secondary exercise group. Also, comparing the exercise dependent groups, primary individuals scored lower on *neuroticism*, *addictiveness* and *impulsiveness* and higher on *extraversion* and *venturesomeness*, than secondary exercise dependent individuals. It is noteworthy that it was the combination of exercise dependence and eating disorders (i.e. a double dependency) that produced the highest scores of all the four groups on the *addictiveness* personality dimension.

It is also useful to compare these results with those obtained in the Florida study (in spite of differences in the type of samples used (targeted exercisers versus general university students) and a number of limitations associated with the Florida study), as the measures used overlap to a degree. On one hand, the finding that those in the primary group (as well as the secondary and no-dependence exercise groups) were more neurotic than controls tended to confirm the link between primary exercise dependence and high *neuroticism* scores obtained by Hausenblas and Giacobbi (2004). On the other hand, the *extraversion* results, where the primary exercise dependent group scores were no different from the control group scores, seemed to contradict Hausenblas and Giacobbi's (2004) finding that *extraversion* scores were a predictor of primary exercise dependence.

Both studies found that exercise dependence was strongly linked to high scores on *neuroticism* and in the Birmingham study that secondary exercise dependent individuals were significantly more neurotic than the primary exercise dependent participants. This is an interesting finding because of the role that anxiety plays in people with anorexia and bulimia nervosa, discussed in Chapter 4.

However, as Blaydon *et al.* (2002) noted, an additional criticism of the Bamber *et al.* (2000a) study is that the low EDQ cut-off point of 116 used to identify those individuals who were exercise dependent may have allowed some borderline cases to be included. This possibility was acknowledged by Bamber *et al.* (2000b) in their publication on a qualitative analysis of exercise dependence:

> it is possible that the EDQ cut-off criterion we used was insufficiently rigorous and that the primary exercise dependence group included women

who were not truly exercise dependent. Some support for this emerges from the testimonies of Angie and Maureen. Although both met our cut-off criteria on the EDQ, there was no evidence of exercise dependence from their interviews. In addition they displayed no evidence of general psychological distress or morbid personality.

(Bamber *et al.*, 2000b, p. 429)

Thus, although the study produced some interesting findings on the differences among the groups, because of the possibility of misclassification of groups, the results may need to be treated with caution.

Before moving on to describe the Hong Kong studies, it may be useful to point out here that the theoretical background and conceptual thinking behind the personality measures used in the Florida and Birmingham studies are different from those used in the reversal theory-based Hong Kong studies. The NEO-FFI (NEO-PI-R) and EPQ-R are traditional 'trait-type' tests, which measure what are considered to be relatively permanent, consistent personality characteristics. However, in reversal theory the notion of personality is more flexible than the concept of personality traits and allows for the fact that a person's personality has a degree of inconsistency and may change depending on the person's experience and the circumstances pertaining at the time (Apter, 2001). For example, a person may spend time in both the mastery and the sympathy states and reverse between them. However, it is likely that a person will spend more time in one state than the other. That dominant state may be the mastery state, and the fact that more time is spent in the mastery state than the sympathy state in any given period means that he or she is described as *mastery dominant*. This applies to all four metamotivational pairs of states and, taken together, the various dominances are really aggregates of a person's personality characteristics over time (see Appendix A and below). Also, the concept of dominance has been extended recently to distinguish between, for example, dominance in life in general and dominance in specific situations such as the context of sport and exercise activities (Apter, 2001).

The Hong Kong studies

Two reversal theory-based studies were carried out and written up in three journal publications and a PhD thesis (Blaydon, 2001; Blaydon and Lindner, 2002; Blaydon *et al.*, 2002; Blaydon *et al.*, 2004). One study (Blaydon *et al.*, 2004)[1] focused on a sample of highly active amateur sport participants. The sample included male and female international and local participants from a wide range of sport and exercise activities (e.g. distance running, weight training, swimming, aerobics, rugby and hockey). Some participants were recruited by advertisements placed in various international and local sports magazines; others were recruited from various specialized sports clubs and gyms. The sample included participants from elite and non-elite level competitive and recreational sports. All participants exercised for more than four hours a week, as this is thought to be the general criterion for identification of exercise dependence (Ogden *et al.* 1997). With the assistance of the British Eating Disorders Association, an additional group of participants who were clinically classified as having eating disorders was also included to provide a total of 393 male and female respondents.

The participants were assigned to groups using the EDQ and the Eating Attitudes Test (EAT; Garner and Garfinkel, 1979) measures. For the EDQ, cluster analysis and a more stringent criterion for exercise dependence using a cut-off point of 130 (considerably higher than the cut-off point of 116 applied in the Bamber *et al.* (2000a) study) ensured that borderline cases were not included. Those scoring above 130 were classed as exercise dependent and those below 125 as not exercise dependent (the few participants scoring between 125 and 130 were not included in the analysis). The EAT, with the prescribed cut-off point of 30, was used to identify participants with eating disorders. This allowed the participants to be divided into primary exercise dependent (N = 58; high EDQ-low EAT), secondary exercise dependent (N = 52; high EDQ-high EAT), eating disordered (N = 45; low EDQ-high EAT) and control (N = 238; low EDQ-low EAT) groups.

In addition to completing the EDQ and EAT measures, participants provided personal information about gender, main sport participation, hours of exercise and competitive level. To measure the personality profiles of the participants, a slightly modified version of the Motivational Style Profile (MSP; Apter *et al.*, 1998) related to the specific context of sports and exercise known as the Motivational Style Profile for Sports and Exercise (MSP-SE) was used. The questionnaire consists of six dimensions, four based on the metamotivational pairs from reversal theory (*telic-paratelic, negativistic-conformist, autic-alloic, mastery-sympathy*) and two extra pairs (*arousal-avoiding-arousal-seeking* and *optimism-pessimism*). Scoring allows six *dominances* to be derived (see Table 6.2).

Analysis using Multivariate Analysis of Variance (MANOVA) provided some interesting personality differences (Blaydon, 2001; Blaydon *et al.*, 2004). For example, the secondary exercise dependence group was found to score significantly higher on telic and arousal-avoidance dominance in the exercise context than the other groups. This secondary group was also more conformist and less optimism dominant than the primary exercise dependence and no-dependence control groups. The exercise-context dominance pattern for the primary and no-dependence control group was very similar. Only one important difference was found: the control group was more mastery dominant than the primary group. The primary exercise dependence and control groups' telic and arousal-avoidance dominance scores were lower than those of the eating disordered group (see Table 6.3). These differences attest to the fact that primary exercise dependence is a condition that is psychologically distinct from secondary exercise dependence at the amateur level (Blaydon *et al.*, 2004, p. 1428). In addition, they allow personality profiles of

Table 6.2 Reversal theory concepts and corresponding MSP/MSP-SE measures

Metamotivational pairs	Subscales	Characteristics
telic – paratelic	telic	serious-minded, goal-oriented
	paratelic	playful, present-oriented
negativistic – conformist	negativism	rebellious, stubborn
	conformity	compliant, agreeable
autic – alloic	autic	self-centred
	alloic	other-centred
mastery – sympathy	mastery	desire for control, tough
	sympathy	desire for harmony, sensitive
Additional pairs		
arousal-avoiding –	arousal-avoidance	need for relaxation
arousal-seeking	arousal-seeking	need for excitement
optimism – pessimism	optimism	positive outlook
	pessimism	negative outlook

primary and secondary exercise dependent individuals to be constructed. In the exercise context, secondary exercise dependent individuals tend to be more serious and planning oriented, focusing on the achievement of future goals. They prefer to avoid highly arousing activities or situations and to comply with rules and be agreeable. Their attitude to exercise tends to be less optimistic than primary exercise dependent individuals. In contrast, although the profile for primary exercise dependent individuals is similar, they are less serious and focused on planning and achieving future goals in the exercise context than secondary exercise dependent individuals. They also tend not to avoid arousal as much, or be as rule-compliant, cooperative and agreeable as secondary exercise dependent individuals. Their attitude to exercise tends to be more positive than secondary exercise dependent individuals.

The fact that the sample of highly active amateurs in this study covered a wide cross-section of sports and exercise activities may have affected the results to some degree. Research that focuses on a particular sport or group of athletes might provide a clearer picture.

Another Hong Kong study concentrated on a specific sport and targeted competitive triathletes (Blaydon and Lindner, 2002; Blaydon *et al.*, 2002). Participants were recruited at two competitive triathlon events. A total of 203 male and female triathletes from a local competition in Hong Kong (*N* = 70) and the 1998 World Triathlon Championships in Lausanne, Switzerland (*N* = 133) took part in the study. In addition to the EDQ and EAT, participants all completed the standard Motivational Style Profile (MSP; Apter *et al.*, 1998) and answered questions relating to descriptive variables such as age, gender, body mass index (BMI), exercise years, triathlon years, weekly training hours, number of other sports and professional or amateur

Table 6.3 Significant differences in personality characteristics of exercise dependent athletes in highly active amateur sport and exercise participants (MSP-SE; Blaydon, 2001; Blaydon *et al.*, 2004) and triathletes (MSP; Blaydon and Lindner, 2002; Blaydon *et al.*, 2002)

Highly active amateur sport and exercise participants	MSP-SE scores
Telic	Secondary > Eat > Primary, Control
Arousal avoidance	Secondary > Eat > Primary, Control
Conformity	Secondary > Primary, Control
Mastery	Control > Primary, Eat
Optimism	Primary, Control > Eat > Secondary

Triathletes	MSP scores
Telic	Secondary > Primary > Control
Arousal avoidance	Primary, Secondary > Eat, Control
Conformity	Secondary > Eat, Control
Autic	Primary, Secondary > Eat, Control
Mastery	Secondary, Eat > Control
Optimism	Primary, Secondary > Eat

Amateur and professional triathletes	MSP scores
Telic/Arousal avoidance/Autic/Mastery/Optimism	Professional triathletes > Amateur triathletes
Telic/Conformity/Autic/Mastery	Amateur triathletes: Secondary > Primary
Optimism	Amateur triathletes: Primary, Secondary, Control strongly optimism dominant; Eat strongly pessimism dominant
Telic/Arousal avoidance/Conformity/Autic/Mastery/Optimism	Professional triathletes: Primary, Secondary similar on all dominances; similar to Eat on mastery scores

status. Following group classification using the EDQ and the EAT, groups of 52 primary and 37 secondary exercise dependent triathletes, 21 eating disordered participants, and 61 controls were identified. The cut-off point for the EDQ was 135, and 32 triathletes scoring in the middle ranges were eliminated; for the remaining 171, cluster analysis revealed a score of 135 or above. For the EAT, those scoring above 30 were classified as having eating disorders.

Analysis of the descriptive data using MANOVAs and post hoc tests revealed a number of significant differences between groups. For example, the secondary exercise dependence group had significantly lower average BMI than the control group. The primary exercise dependence group had been exercising for significantly more years, and both exercise dependence groups trained for more hours per week than the control group with no dependence. No important differences were found between the exercise dependence groups and the eating disordered group on these variables (Blaydon and Lindner, 2002).

With regard to personality data, the main part of the analysis was aimed at identifying differences among the four groups of triathletes as a whole and differences between professional and amateur triathletes within those groups. When the four triathlete groups were compared, MANOVAs with follow-up tests resulted in highly significant main effects for groups in dominances, and interactions between group and status (professional or amateur) were also generally significant. The two exercise dependence groups had personality profiles that were significantly more arousal-avoiding and autic dominant than the other groups, and more optimism dominant than the eating disordered group. In addition, the secondary exercise dependence group was significantly more conformist dominant than the eating disordered and control groups. Also, the secondary group (along with the eating disordered group) was significantly more mastery dominant than the control group. Only one personality dimension was found that distinguished between the primary and secondary exercise dependence groups in this sport-specific sample of triathletes. The secondary group was found to be more telic dominant than the primary group, and both groups were more telic dominant than the control group. This result replicates the telic dominance findings in the Hong Kong study of highly active amateurs. However, in this triathlete study, the primary and secondary exercise dependence groups' profiles matched in terms of arousal avoidance, autic and optimism dominance.

In comparison with the control group's profile, the secondary exercise dependence group differed significantly from controls on five dominances (optimism was the exception) and the primary group on three out of six (telic, arousal-avoidance, autic dominance) (see Table 6.3). Compared to normal controls, secondary exercise dependent athletes are more serious and goal oriented, more compliant, more self-focused; they have a greater need to be in control, and a greater need to avoid unnecessary arousal. Similarly, compared to controls, primary exercise dependent athletes are also more serious and goal oriented and more self-focused, and they have a greater need to avoid unnecessary arousal.

When professional and amateur triathletes were compared, in general professionals had significantly higher scores than the amateur triathletes for all dominances except conformity. However, when the status (professional/ amateur) of triathletes was entered into the analysis as an independent variable, the differences between the primary and secondary amateur triathletes were pronounced. The amateur secondary exercise dependent triathletes were significantly more telic, conformist, autic and mastery dominant than the amateur primary exercise dependent triathletes. The amateur triathlete exercise dependence and control groups were strongly optimism dominant, while the amateur triathlete eating disordered group showed marked pessimism dominance. The professional triathlete primary and secondary group participants were very similar and both groups were similar to the professional triathlete eating disordered group on mastery dominance scores.

It is interesting that clear differences in personality profiles between professional and amateur triathletes were demonstrated. It may be that the stronger dominance profile in professionals as compared to their amateur counterparts played a role in their successful progression to professional status (Blaydon *et al.*, 2002). They may be prepared to do more to achieve that status; for example, professional triathletes were found to train for significantly more hours per week, and had lower BMIs than amateur triathletes (Blaydon and Lindner, 2002).

It is also interesting that within each of the professional and amateur sub-samples, distinctive dominance patterns between the exercise dependence groups and the controls and eating disordered groups were again identified. This pattern was strongest for professional primary and secondary exercise dependence groups, whose scores were similar and included the full palette of telic, conformist, autic, mastery, arousal-avoiding and optimism dominances.

Kerr (1997) predicted that the exercise dependent individual's motivational style profile was likely to be telic-conformist-autic-mastery. The results of the Hong Kong studies seem to suggest that his prediction was generally correct. However, the results for triathletes (especially professionals) also show that arousal-avoidance and possibly optimism dominance may well need to be added. Further, the personality characteristics associated with these dominances may also be necessary for exercise dependence.

Certainly, seriously committing oneself to training regularly in compliance with planned training schedules; achieving personal goals in terms of training duration, speed of performance or distances covered; relishing challenges and constantly pushing one's body and enduring discomfort and pain; being generally egoistic and concerned with oneself and one's own performance; having self-control and commitment, while being positive about the future; and being a tough and strong competitor who badly wants to win when competing against others are characteristics associated with high level athletes (e.g. Hardy *et al.*, 1996; Hemery, 1986; Orlick, 1986).

Closing comments

It has long been thought by psychologists that personality is shaped by both genetic influences inherited from parents and environmental influences through the early stages of a person's life span. These influences are thought to be interrelated. Therefore, it seems plausible that the motivational profile characteristics exhibited by exercise dependent people are the result of their parents' genes but also of their experience of sport and exercise activities during childhood through the adolescent years and into adulthood. Their inherited characteristics and their pleasant (or unpleasant) experience will attract them to (or drive them away from) the particular types of activities associated with exercise addiction (e.g. endurance sports). If the attraction leads to participation and it endures for long enough, it will help to mould the personalities of, for example, exercise dependent triathletes. However, to what extent people are liable to become exercise dependent because of their personality makeup, or how much they develop the typical exercise dependent motivational dominance profile in the process of becoming addicted to exercising, remains an intriguing issue.

In the introduction to this chapter, attention was drawn to Brown's (1997) Hedonic Management Model of Addiction and his argument that individual differences in personality might make some people more vulnerable to becoming addicted to substances and activities than others. If this is correct, how does the exercise dependent person's motivational profile make them vulnerable, especially with reference to the telic, conformist and arousal-avoidant dominances identified in both Hong Kong studies? Brown's (1997) suggestion was that the hedonic gap (the discrepancy between the level of negative feeling states a person can tolerate and the level they experience) might be greater in people with certain personality types. One possible explanation is, therefore, that the exercise dependent people in the Hong Kong studies, who have a strong preference for low arousal in general and who want to avoid anxiety-provoking high arousal situations in life as much as possible, often have a mismatch in the level of arousal they prefer and the level that they actually feel or experience. For them exercise may have become the most effective way of manipulating arousal and hedonic tone and reducing the discrepancy between felt and preferred levels of arousal, in the way that Brown (1997) proposed. In other words, exercise is 'what works for them' as a means of dealing with the uncomfortable levels of heightened arousal and anxiety that are at variance with their personality profile and preferences, and this is what gets them 'hooked' (see Chapter 3).

It follows that reversals could also help to reduce the hedonic gap in an exercise dependent exerciser whose personality profile made him or her vulnerable to that addiction. Exercise could be used to induce or facilitate reversals to other states, so that, for example, unpleasant anxiety as a result of high arousal in the telic state could be re-interpreted in the paratelic state as pleasant excitement. In addition to changing an unpleasant emotion into a pleasant one, this change would also serve to match up felt and preferred levels of arousal and provide relief as long as the reversal to the paratelic state was maintained. This could also lead to reliance on exercise as a means to induce reversals and, over time, to an addiction to the activity

Chapter 6 examined some of the available evidence on exercise dependence and personality obtained using quantitative research methods and questionnaires administered to large groups of people. These quantitative studies provided a broad, but relatively unfocused picture of the similarities and differences in personality between the various exercise dependent and other groups. Chapter 7 will be approached from the qualitative side of the methodological coin, using a more individual approach. The results of semi-structured interviews will be used to provide a deeper, more detailed picture of exercise dependent and eating disordered people and how they perceive their dependencies.

Note

1   Readers should note that an uncorrected proof of the Blaydon *et al.* (2004) manuscript was inadvertently published in the journal. This regrettable and rather embarrassing occurrence has meant that several of the results correctly listed in Blaydon's (2001) PhD thesis are incorrectly stated in the journal article. In cases of doubt please contact the authors for clarification.

References

Apter, M. J. (ed.) (2001) *Motivational styles in everyday life: A guide to reversal theory*, Washington DC: American Psychological Association.

Apter, M. J., Mallows, R. and Williams, S. (1998) 'The development of the Motivational Style Profile', *Personality and Individual Differences*, 24, 7–18.

Bamber, D., Cockerill, I. M. and Carroll, D. (2000a) 'The pathological status of exercise dependence', *British Journal of Sports Medicine*, 34, 125–32.

Bamber, D., Cockerill, I. M., Rodgers, S. and Carroll, D. (2000b) '"It's exercise or nothing": A qualitative analysis of exercise dependence', *British Journal of Sports Medicine*, 34, 423–30.

Bamber, D., Cockerill, I. M., Rodgers, S. and Carroll, D. (2003) 'Diagnostic criteria for exercise dependence in women', *British Journal of Sports Medicine*, 37, 393–400.

Blaydon, M. J. (2001) *Descriptive and metamotivational characteristics of primary and secondary exercise dependent and eating disordered participants in intense physical activity*, unpublished doctoral dissertation, Hong Kong: The University of Hong Kong.

Blaydon, M. J. and Lindner, K. J. (2002) 'Eating disorders and exercise dependence in triathletes', *Eating Disorders*, 10, 49–60.

Blaydon, M. J., Lindner, K. J. and Kerr, J. H. (2002) 'Metamotivational characteristics of eating-disordered and exercise-dependent triathletes', *Psychology of Sport and Exercise*, 3, 223–36.

Blaydon, M. J., Lindner, K. J. and Kerr, J. H. (2004) 'Metamotivational characteristics of exercise dependence and eating disorders in highly active amateur sport participants', *Personality and Individual Differences*, 36, 1419–32.

Brown, R. I. F. (1997) 'A theoretical model of behavioural addictions – Applied to offending', in J. E. Hodge, M. McMurran and C. R. Hollin (eds) *Addicted to crime?*, New York: Wiley, 13–65.

Cockerill, I. M. and Riddington, M. E. (1996) 'Exercise dependence and associated disorders: A review', *Counselling Psychology Quarterly*, 9, 119–29.

Costa, P. T. and McCrae, R. R. (1992a) *Revised NEO Personality Inventory (NEO-PI-R) and NEO Five-Factor Inventory (NEO-FFI) professional manual*, Odessa FL: Psychological Assessment Resources.

Costa, P. T. and McCrae, R. R. (1992b) *The NEO-PI-R: Professional manual*, Odessa FL: Psychological Assessment Resources.

Eysenck, H. J. and Eysenck, S. B. G. (1991) *Manual of the Eysenck Personality Scales*, London: Hodder & Staunton.

Fairburn, C. G. and Beglin, S. J. (1994) 'Assessment of eating disorders: Interview or self-report questionnaire?', *International Journal of Eating Disorders*, 16, 363–70.

Garner, D. M. (1991) *Eating Disorder Inventory-2 manual*, Odessa FL: Psychological Assessment Resources.

Garner, D. M. and Garfinkel, P. E. (1979) 'The Eating Attitudes Test: An index of the symptoms of anorexia nervosa', *Psychological Medicine*, 9, 273–9.

Godin, G. and Shephard, R. (1985) 'A simple method to assess exercise behaviour in the community', *Canadian Journal of Applied Sport Science*, 10, 141–6.

Goldberg, D. and Williams, P. (1988) *A user's guide to the General Health Questionnaire*, Windsor, Berkshire: NFER-Nelson.

Hardy, L., Jones, G. and Gould, D. (1996) *Understanding psychological preparation for sport: Theory and practice of elite performers*, Chichester: Wiley.

Hausenblas, H. A. and Symons Downs D. (2002a) 'Exercise dependence: A systematic review', *Psychology of Sport and Exercise*, 3, 89–123.

Hausenblas, H. A. and Symons Downs, D. (2002b) 'How much is too much? The development and validation of the Exercise Dependence Scale', *Psychology and Health*, 17, 387–404.

Hausenblas, H. A. and Giacobbi, P. R. (2004) 'Relationship between exercise dependence symptoms and personality', *Personality and Individual Differences*, 36, 1265–73.

Hemery, D. (1986) *The pursuit of sporting excellence: A study of sport's highest achievers*, London: Willow Books.

Kerr, J. H. (1997) *Motivation and emotion in sport: Reversal theory*, Hove: Psychology Press.

Loumidis, K. S. and Wells, A. (1998) 'Assessment of beliefs in excessive exercise: The development and preliminary validation of the Exercise Beliefs Questionnaire', *Personality and Individual Differences*, 25, 553–67.

Ogden, J., Veale, D. M. W. and Summers, Z. (1997) 'The development and validation of the Exercise Dependence Questionnaire', *Addiction Research*, 5, 343–56.

Orlick, T. (1986) *Psyching for sport: Mental training for athletes*, Champaign IL: Leisure Press/Human Kinetics.

Paa, H. K. and Larson, L. M. (1998) 'Predicting level of restrained eating behaviour in adult women', *International Journal of Eating Disorders*, 24, 91–4.

Rosenberg, M. (1965) *Society and the adolescent self-image*, Princeton NJ: Princeton University Press.

Veale, D. (1995) 'Does primary exercise dependence really exist?', in J. Annett, B. Cripps and H. Steinberg (eds) *Exercise addiction: Motivation for participation in sport and exercise*, Leicester: The British Psychological Society, 1–5.

7   'Can't do without my exercise'

What exercise dependent people say about themselves and their dependency

The advantage of qualitative over quantitative research is that it allows much more detailed information to be obtained about a person's experience and motivation. For example, in qualitative research based on interviews, the essence of the procedure with face-to-face interaction is generally more personal than is possible in quantitative research and allows the interviewer to follow up on interesting or unexpected points raised during the interview. Interviews can sometimes encounter or deal with difficult material that might be threatening or unpleasant for the interviewee, which, if handled sensitively, can provide greater insight into a person's feelings, experience and behaviour than would be revealed by the completion of a questionnaire.

There have been at least four studies in which the researchers adopted a qualitative approach and undertook in-depth interviews with exercisers. The first was the pioneering research work involving 'obligatory' runners carried out by psychiatrist Yates and her colleagues at the University of Arizona in the US (Yates, 1991; Yates et al., 1983). Three other more recent research studies have taken a combined qualitative and quantitative approach, relying on exercise dependence and eating disorder questionnaires such as the EDQ (Ogden et al., 1997) and the EAT (Garner and Garfinkel, 1979) to separate out individuals who were exercise dependent and/or had eating disorders, followed by interviews with the participants.

Bamber and colleagues carried out an interview study, published in two separate papers (Bamber et al., 2000b, 2003), as part of the Birmingham group's work on exercise dependence described in the previous chapter. Cox and Orford (2004), based in Shrewsbury, England, undertook an interview study of 'people who could be labelled as addicted to exercise'. The final study was an additional feature of the Hong Kong quantitative research described in Chapter 6, which included the collection of interview data (Blaydon, 2001). The results of these qualitative studies will be described and examined in detail in this chapter.

The Arizona interview study

Yates and her team (Yates, 1991; Yates et al., 1983) undertook in-depth interviews with more than 150 male and female runners who ran an average of more than 50 miles per week. These runners were recruited at a sports medicine clinic, at races and through other runners. Many were middle-aged high achievers who enjoyed running because it made them feel better and contributed to their emotional balance.

Among these runners, the researchers identified several whom they labelled 'obligatory' runners. For these participants, running had become a central feature of their lives, to the extent that they continued to run even when injured and seemed to be unable to do without running. The researchers identified a number of similarities between obligatory runners and eating disordered women, including commitment to exercise or dieting; attempting to control the body through exercise or dieting; spending most of their free time engaged in or thinking about exercise and diet; investing emotionally in exercise or dieting (to the extent that these become more intense and important than investing in family or work); causing damage to the body through extremes of exercise or dieting; and experiencing withdrawal symptoms when prevented from exercising or dieting (Yates, 1991).

The researchers chose to label the runners that were interviewed as 'obligatory' or 'compulsive' runners rather than 'addicted to' or 'dependent on' running, pointing out that they were healthy and not pathological (Yates, 1991). However careful reading of the cases from the interviews presented by Yates (1991) indicates that the symptoms of obligatory running and the symptoms exhibited by exercise dependent runners described elsewhere (e.g. Szabo, 2000; Veale, 1995) are very similar. Also, the differences between obligatory and non-obligatory runners are very similar to the differences between exercise dependent runners and runners without exercise dependence. As noted by Yates (1991):

> The non-obligatory runners differ from the obligatory runners in that they do not build their lives around running; they continue to enjoy many other activities. They are not as rigid in their training or as extreme in their self-expectations. They seldom think about running when they are otherwise engaged. They are more sociable and less likely to run alone. When they are sick or hurt, they stop or cut down on their running. Most of the differences between obligatory and non-obligatory are a matter of degree, rather than kind.
>
> (Yates, 1991, p. 30)

Many of the runners interviewed in Yates (1991) were concerned about weight and diet, and used running to make their dieting more effective. There were two ways in which this could work:

> When emaciated runners progressively increase their running and dieting so that they can diminish, even further, their percentage of body fat, they could be said to be following an anorexic format. When they counter the amount of food they consume by boosting the distance they run so

that they will not gain weight, they could be said to be following a bulimic format. In both formats, the need for absolute control of the body is similar to that found in the eating disorders.

(Yates, 1991, p. 43)

Not only was this study one of the first, if not the first in the field that used qualitative methods but it also established the link between intense exercise, eating disorders and associated mental problems.

The Birmingham interview study

Bamber *et al.* (2000b, 2003) adopted a qualitative approach involving a social constructionist revision of grounded theory (e.g. Glaser and Strauss, 1967) also used, for example, by Charmaz (1990). Rather than basing the concepts that account for people's interpretations of their experiences on established theory, grounded theory takes the view that conceptual developments should come from qualitative data. However, Bamber *et al.* (2000b) decided that because they had the results from their quantitative study (Bamber *et al.*, 2000a), adopting a social constructionist revision of the grounded theory approach would be more appropriate than the original approach. Bamber *et al.* (2000b, p. 424) thought that this approach 'would enable the researchers to test ideas about exercise dependence based on their previous quantitative analysis, while remaining open to the emergence and exploration of new themes as they arise from the data'. The purpose of this study was to use semi-structured interviews to examine exercise dependence in order to formulate diagnostic criteria.

The general methodology used in the Birmingham research was described in the previous chapter (Bamber *et al.*, 2000a). The additional qualitative data was collected from sub-samples from the main participant cohort of females involved in physically active sports, dance or exercise used in the quantitative study. This sub-sample took part in semi-structured interviews consisting of the Eating Disorders Examination (EDE; Fairburn and Cooper, 1993) and the Exercise Dependence Interview (EXDI) developed by the authors in a format similar to the EDE. The order of administration of EDE and EXDI was counterbalanced. Prior to the interview, participants also completed the Exercise Dependence Questionnaire (EDQ; Ogden *et al.*, 1997).

The EXDI was based on information from a number of sources, including Veale's (1995) exercise dependence criteria, APA substance dependence criteria (DSM-IV; American Psychiatric Association, 1994), general exercise dependence and eating disorder literature, and available questionnaire measures of exercise dependence. It was designed to examine: exercise behaviour for the previous three months; exercise cognitions; aspects of exercise dependence as a behavioural pathology; reputed characteristics of exercise dependence; effects of being unable to exercise on eating attitudes and behaviours; temporal relationships between exercise and eating or dieting behaviour; the individual's own perceptions of exercise dependence; and the history of psychological illness and treatment (Bamber *et al.*, 2000b, 2003).

Interviews were conducted by a trained interviewer who obtained written consent before tape recording the one- to three-hour interviews. A number of rigorous procedures were used to ensure the accuracy of participants' recollections within a correct time frame. In addition, debriefing of any participants who disclosed disordered eating attitudes and behaviours took place, and participants were allowed to ask questions about the research. The interviewer also made post-interview notes on her thoughts and ideas about each interview (Bamber *et al.*, 2000b, 2003).

Once the interviews were transcribed verbatim, participants' responses to the EDE coded, and eating disorder diagnoses completed, the usual procedures for safeguarding the analysis of qualitative data were followed. These included inter-rater reliability checks and the writing of a précis for each interview. Information on demographic data, core diagnostic features of eating disorders and exercise dependence, the chronology of eating and/or dieting and sport and/or exercise involvement, and the history of psychological illness and treatment were also included as part of a summary sheet. The QSR NUD*IST 4.0 (1993) software package was used to 'sort' the raw data statements from the interview transcripts, post-interview journal entries and summary sheets into first-order themes, then second-order themes, then general dimensions. Examples of raw data statements included 'It's exercise or nothing'; 'My exercise is my social life, I don't have a social life outside that'; 'It has a tendency to creep up'; and 'There aren't many people in my front room at 5.00 am' (Bamber *et al.*, 2000b, p. 395). First-order themes included *anxiety, depression, injury, salience of exercising over other activities, lying about exercising, regulation of emotions* and *feeling in control*. There were eleven second-order themes (e.g. *social and occupational, physical, exercise behaviour, tolerance*) and four general dimensions (*impaired functioning, withdrawal, associated features* and *presence of an eating disorder*). The results of the study were published in two papers: the first examined the comments of 16 participants from the sub-sample of 56 (Bamber *et al.*, 2000b); the second examined the responses of the 56 participants as a whole (Bamber *et al.*, 2003).

Bamber et al. (2000b)

In the Bamber *et al.* (2000b) qualitative paper, 16 participants (four participants from each group: primary and secondary exercise dependent, eating disordered, and exercisers with no dependence) were selected and interviewed. Information on how they were selected was not provided. Classification of participants was based on their scores on the EDQ (cut-off point 116) and the Eating Disorder Examination Questionnaire (EDE-Q; Fairburn and Beglin, 1994). Interviews subsequently confirmed that all eight participants from the secondary exercise dependence and eating disorder groups had eating disorders and that participants in the group with only an eating disorder were not exercise dependent.

In their results section the authors presented detailed commentaries on the individuals within each group, backed up by a selection of quotes from the relevant participants. The authors concluded that where exercise dependence was found among the participants it was always in the presence of an eating disorder and that there was no evidence of primary exercise dependence. Psychological distress was found only in secondary exercise dependent individuals and in those who only had an eating disorder. However, the descriptions in the Bamber et al. (2000b) paper indicate that the four interviewees identified as primary exercise dependent were misclassified. Two of these, who had previously failed to meet the EDE-Q criterion for eating disorders adopted in this research, disclosed at interview that they did have eating disorders. One, a track and field athelete, had an eating problem associated with restricting her weight for her event while the second was anorexic. The other two interviewees had EDQ scores too low to categorize them safely in the primary group. The authors acknowledged the failure to classify participants correctly and the problems associated with the low EDQ cut-off point (see also Chapter 6) as one reason for not finding evidence of primary exercise dependence. Identifying misclassifications is one of the advantages of the qualitative approach, which allows researchers to go beyond the more superficial level of questionnaires.

Bamber et al. (2003)

In the Bamber et al. (2003) paper, 56 exercisers were interviewed with a view to formulating diagnostic criteria for exercise dependence. Of the 56, 42 showed no symptoms of exercise dependence or problem exercising, ten met the criteria for secondary exercise dependence and the remaining four exhibited problem exercising, but could not be diagnosed as exercise dependent. There were no exercisers classified as primary exercise dependent. These diagnoses were based on a comparison of participants' responses with Bamber et al.'s (2003) new criteria for secondary exercise dependence (see below and Table 7.1).

The results section first concentrated on each of the four general dimensions identified through QSR NUD*IST (1993) analysis procedures. These were: *impaired functioning, withdrawal, associated features* and *presence of an eating disorder.* The authors dealt with each in turn, describing what was included in each dimension and providing examples from the interview transcripts. Diagnosis of exercise dependence required evidence of problems in at least two of these areas and confirmation involving a further review of the evidence by one of the researchers, who was a qualified clinical psychologist.

Impaired functioning was concerned with serious psychological, social and occupational, physical and behavioural dysfunction. Examples of impaired psychological functioning, which, the researchers found, occurred only when exercise became all consuming, were inability to concentrate as a result of thinking about exercise, exercise-induced fatigue and conflict with partner, family and friends.

Two main themes emerged under the general dimension of *withdrawal*, which the researchers labelled a 'clinically significant adverse response to a change in or interruption of exercise habits' and 'evidence of a persistent desire and/or unsuccessful efforts to control or reduce exercise' (Bamber *et al.*, 2003, p. 396). The adverse response often involved negative emotional responses in the form of anxiety, depression, anger or guilt. For example, Peta stated:

> I was mad at myself, I felt really angry, I couldn't concentrate on anything and I felt moody and aggressive. I was really sarcastic with my husband and I felt like a big fat blob. Oh it was a dreadful day, I just felt so agitated and so out of control. It was a rotten time, and the other time when I couldn't I felt angry at that person, I felt angry at everyone because I couldn't go and get my hour in the gym or a swim and just like, less interested, just not interested in anything.
>
> (Bamber *et al.*, 2003, p. 396)

Unsuccessful efforts to control exercise sometimes involved fantasizing about giving up or cutting down on exercise but not being able to do so. For instance, Anne, a secondary exercise dependent individual, stated:

> I think it's a dream that I would love to be able to do at one point in the future but at the moment I would not be able to, no way . . . I try to cut down but I know that I won't.
>
> (Bamber *et al.*, 2003, p. 396)

The *associated features* dimension included increasing tolerance for exercise, increases in exercise volume, solitary and/or daily exercising, being deceptive about exercising and exercising primarily to control weight and body shape. These were classed by the researchers as 'associated features' or 'useful pointers' because they were not shown to be clear diagnostic features of exercise dependence:

> Although intentionally increasing exercise levels was a common practice, tolerance cannot be inferred from this behaviour. Accordingly tolerance was not included as a diagnostic criterion . . . A key finding in the present study was the importance of cognitions, such as ruminations about, or inflexible attitudes towards, exercising, as signifiers of exercise dependence. In contrast, frequency, duration or overall volume of exercise undertaken did not differentiate unambiguously dependent and non-dependent exercisers.
>
> (Bamber *et al.*, 2003, p. 398)

The fourth general dimension, the *presence or absence of an eating disorder*, was based on participants' responses to EDE questions. Eighteen were found to have eating disorders, and an additional nine interviewees had non-clinical eating behaviour and attitude problems.

Based on their analysis of these 56 female exercisers' interview narratives, Bamber *et al.* (2003) proposed a new set of criteria for secondary exercise dependence (see Table 7.1). The researchers recommended that 'impairments in two or more of four areas of functioning and withdrawal in either or both of its manifestations strongly intimated pathology and, accordingly, provided appropriate diagnostic criteria for exercise dependence' (Bamber *et al.*, 2003, p. 397).

Table 7.1 New diagnostic criteria for secondary exercise dependence

---

The following three criteria are necessary for a diagnosis of secondary exercise dependence:

1. Impaired functioning*

   The individual shows evidence of impaired functioning in at least two of the following areas:
   a. Psychological – e.g. ruminations or intrusive thoughts about exercise, salience of thoughts about exercise, anxiety, or depression
   b. Social and occupational – e.g. salience of exercising above all social activities, inability to work
   c. Physical – e.g. exercising causes or aggravates health or injury yet continues to exercise when medically contraindicated
   d. Behavioural – e.g. stereotyped and inflexible behaviour

2. Withdrawal

   The individual shows evidence of one or more of the following:
   a. Clinically significant adverse response to a change or interruption of exercise habits. Response may be physical, psychological, social, or behavioural, e.g. severe anxiety or depression, social withdrawal, self harm**
   b. Persistent desire and/or unsuccessful efforts to control or reduce exercise

3. Presence of an eating disorder***

   Associated features
   The following features are indicative but not definitive:
   i. Tolerance – i.e. increasing volumes of exercising required
   ii. High volumes of exercising and/or exercising at least once daily
   iii. Solitary exercising
   iv. Deception – e.g. lying about exercise volume, exercising in secret
   v. Insight – e.g. denial that exercising is a problem

---

*   Exercise is unreasonably salient and/or stereotyped even when considered in appropriate context – e.g. individual is a competitive athlete
** If individual had not abstained from exercise, or would refuse to do so, rate withdrawal according to anticipated response
*** For a diagnosis of primary exercise dependence, all criteria may be the same as for secondary exercise dependence except for the absence, rather than presence, of an eating disorder

Source: Bamber *et al.* 2003. Copyright BMJ Publishing Group Ltd. Reproduced with permission

Previous efforts at describing exercise dependence criteria have been generally constructed from the criteria for other dependencies (e.g. Hausenblas and Symons Downs, 2002; Veale, 1995; see Chapter 1). The advantage of these new diagnostic criteria for secondary exercise dependence is that they are based directly on data from exercise-dependent individuals. Bamber *et al.* (2003) also suggested (even though there were no primary exercise dependent exercisers in their sample) that, although requiring further systematic investigation, the same criteria could be used to diagnose primary exercise dependence in the absence of an eating disorder.

The Shrewsbury interview study

Cox and Orford (2004) set out to examine whether addiction or elements of addiction were present in those who qualified as primary exercise dependent under Veale's (1995) criteria, and whether there was a valid case for the pathological label 'addiction' to be applied to high frequency exercise. The study utilized the original grounded theory approach (e.g. Henwood, 1996; Strauss and Corbin, 1990) to analyse data. This was somewhat similar to the approach used in the Birmingham study. Cox and Orford (2004) were interested in examining the meaning of exercise to people who could be labelled as being exercise dependent and trying to develop a theory from an analysis of their responses. This was perhaps a surprising choice for a research approach given Orford's (2001) well-developed Social-Behavioural-Cognitive-Moral Model of Excessive Appetites (see Chapter 2), but as the authors stated:

> In the case of high frequency exercise the field has been dominated by biomedical and behavioural models. We wanted to distance ourselves from these assumptions and ground a theory in the words and meanings expressed by the participants.
>
> (Cox and Orford, 2004, p. 169)

Cox and Orford (2004) used a 'snowballing' method to recruit volunteer participants. Initially, three people involved in sport and exercise distributed sets of 'recruitment packs' directed at people who exercised six or more hours per week. A total of 70 packs were distributed through eight snowballing routes and 60 were returned. The packs contained a letter and consent form and the EDQ and EAT measures. The participants selected for interview had to be heavily involved in exercise and score 113 or over on the EDQ (a cut-off point even lower than the 116 used in the Birmingham studies) and below 30 on the EAT. Those 12 participants who met these criteria were considered to be exercise dependent, but not anorexic (i.e. primary exercise dependent in Veale's (1995) terms). From this sub-group, five men and five women agreed to be interviewed.

Participants' ages ranged between 23 and 57 years and they had been involved in exercise activities for periods of 18 months to 30 years. These activities were running, cycling, weight training, golf, martial arts, walking, skiing, swimming, canoeing, tennis, squash and aerobics, and all participants were involved in at least two of the activities. The analysis followed procedures described by Charmaz (1995), which were broadly similar to the procedures used in the Birmingham study: (a) initial coding of transcribed tapes; (b) re-examination and subsequent combining of initial codes into focused codes; (c) re-examination and subsequent collapsing of focused codes into categories with shared properties; (d) use of interviewees' words as codes and their phrases as representative of the meaning of categories (e.g. *creating the shape*, *scratching the itch*); (e) continuous memo writing throughout the process; and (f) constant review and comparison of data along with theoretical sampling of new information to develop emerging theory. In an illustration of how this process worked, examples of initial codes such as *controlling mood, pushing self, having routine* were collected into the focused codes *psychological control*, *physical control* and *external control*, and these three focused codes were then collapsed to form a category called *exercising control*. Four other categories that emerged from the analysis were *creating the shape*, *the pay-off*, *the price to pay*, and *scratching an itch or setting a goal*. Each of these categories is discussed in more detail below with illustrative quotes from the participants' transcripts.

The *exercising control* category comprised three different elements: control over the body, control over body image and control through self-imposed structures and routines. As indicated by Cathy's quote, the *exercising control* category involved both psychological and physical aspects of control and these often overlapped:

> the combination of knowing you have that control mentally to push yourself, I suppose to a certain degree you've got control over your body . . . I suppose I am back to the control element again because whilst I was ill and my back was in so much pain I didn't know what was going to happen. I had no real control over how my body was going to respond and what I was going to do, but afterwards, when I could exercise, I'd got that control back again.
>
> (Cox and Orford, 2004, p. 175–6)

The combination of physical and psychological factors was also apparent in the two other elements in the *exercising control* category, control over body image and control through self-imposed structures and routines.

Creating the shape was concerned with individually specific perceptions of developing a particular body shape or image. This was a prominent theme that varied in importance among the interviewees, but all indicated that changing their body shape played some role and acted as a long-term goal, providing motivation and reinforcement for exercising. Cox and Orford (2004) found that all the participants had an ideal image of what they wanted their bodies to look like and used measurement to check progress. Their self-confidence improved and they felt good as they progressed toward their ideal, but at the same time they were fearful of losing the gains that they had made if forced to stop exercising. The ideal body shape differed between men and women. According to the researchers, women wanted to develop and maintain a body shape that made them feel content and physically strong, while men wanted to create a shape that would be impressive to others. For example, Cathy said:

> I know how I want to look and feel, and how looking a certain way makes me feel, so I think it's more just for me ... I'm very critical of my own body I know that. If I were to describe a perfect body image it would be thin it would be fit ... reasonably defined muscles;

while Ben stated:

> I just want the perfect physique really ... just to be well toned ... to have a nice six-pack ... just to look good ... I'd like for people to look and think, 'yeah he looks good'.
> (Cox and Orford, 2004, p. 179)

The pay-off category referred to long-term benefits in improved health, fitness, confidence and general well-being, as well as short-term benefits in mood regulation during and after exercise. As Cox and Orford (2004) pointed out, this included participants' perceptions that *exercising control* and *creating the shape* were positive aspects of their exercising, providing predominantly long-term benefits. Other pay-offs reported by participants were concerned with enhancing mood as a means of, for example, releasing frustration or coping with day-to-day stress. Two examples from the interview transcripts illustrate short-term benefits obtained during an exercise session (Gill) and post-exercise (Henry):

> Gill – There's a point when you start off when I don't want to do it and it hurts and I can't see the point in doing it, particularly if I am feeling depressed but ... you know you warm up, you have a bit of a stretch, you set off again and there's a point where ... it's not like a switch turns from on and off, it's more like a volume control and it slowly gets to feel better and better and better ...
>
> Henry – There is a feeling of physical well-being after working very very hard ... once you've had a shower and relaxed there's a glow about that, a bit of smugness, a bit of self satisfaction ... I enjoy it ... I love it.
> (Cox and Orford, 2004, p. 182)

The price to pay category was concerned with negative aspects of high frequency exercising. It also involved both physical and psychological factors associated with exercise, such as exercising when ill or injured or with long-term injuries, a fear of not being able to exercise, and a negative mood that occurred when the participants were unable to exercise. Exercising when ill or injured was common to all the participants and most accepted that there would be a price to pay later for their heavy involvement in exercising. For example, one participant (Cathy) reported an incident when she played her sport while injured:

> I've torn a muscle in my leg which was quite painful . . . I did it on Tuesday and played hockey on the Saturday, with it strapped, and it was really painful, I could hardly run but I just carried on.
> (Cox and Orford, 2004, p. 183)

Another participant (Fred) stated:

> You try and keep fit and something else gets you in the end . . . I'm sure in later life I'll probably have arthritis and lord knows what because it seem [sic] that sportsmen get trouble with their joints don't they . . . I don't think I'll be walking around like him (father-in-law) when I'm 82.
> (Cox and Orford, 2004, p. 183)

A third participant (Denise) described her emotional reaction and hedonic tone when she had not exercised: 'If I don't train I'm niggly (irritable) and I'm miserable and I feel guilty and horrible and my day just falls to bits' (Cox and Orford, 2004, p. 183). According to Cox and Orford (2004), most exercisers thought that the positive benefits of exercise outweighed the possible negative consequences. They knew and accepted the risks involved and felt that they had achieved the correct balance between enjoying those benefits and paying the price.

The final category *scratching an itch or setting a goal* emerged during the analysis procedure and overlapped with some of the previous categories. It concerned two coexisting parallel or even opposite notions of exercise. These were exercise as an end in itself, catering to short-term pleasurable needs and exercise as a means to an end, producing a long-term goal or aim. It was noted by the authors from the material collected during the interviews that both were equally important and they reported that:

> Some very clear short term itch scratching was described to get the pleasure of the buzz, the heightened mood, the satisfaction and the sense of achievement. An enjoyment of playing/performing exercise was clear throughout the interviews as noted above in the 'pay off' category. Yet, evidence for the constant aiming for the goal was equally strong. This was seen mainly in the creating a shape and exercising control categories. It was also demonstrated in the desire to be fit and healthy alongside goals such as competing and improving at one's chosen

exercise/sport. This demonstrates that neither scratching the itch or goal setting are exclusive when viewing high frequency exercisers.

(Cox and Orford, 2004, p. 184)

It is perhaps disappointing that the Shrewsbury study did not explore in more depth the conflicts that can occur between exercisers and family members or at work, as both Orford's (2001) and Brown's (1997) models emphasized the role that social factors play in addictions and the conflict that can arise as a result. This aspect was included in the Birmingham study under the category *impaired functioning* and included conflict in relationships, social isolation or withdrawal, and work problems. In general there is no clear match between the categories from the Birmingham and Shrewsbury studies, but there is partial overlap. For example, the Birmingham study's *withdrawal* and *associated features* categories could include the Shrewsbury study's *pay the price* and *creating the shape categories respectively*. However, taking into account the different types of exercise dependence being investigated, it is perhaps not surprising that the categories that emerged were somewhat different.

The Hong Kong interview study

Blaydon (2001) adopted a different approach for categorizing interview data. In this case, reversal theory was used to examine participants' comments. A total of seventeen participants from the original sample of 393 in the quantitative Hong Kong study of highly active amateur exercisers (Blaydon et al., 2004; see Chapter 6) agreed to take part in follow-up interviews (Blaydon, 2001). From these seventeen participants a sub-sample of nine participants (six males, three females), representing a spread of participants across all four groups, was chosen for analysis. Prior to interview the participants had been placed in the four participant groups from their scores on the EDQ (cut-off point 130) and EAT (prescribed cut-off point 30) measures (Blaydon et al., 2004): primary exercise dependence, two males; secondary exercise dependence, two females; eating disorder only, one female; and no dependence, four males. In each case, motivational style dominance scores relating to sport and exercise (MSP-SE; Apter et al., 1998; Blaydon et al., 2004) were available for each interviewee, as were individual Body Mass Index (BMI) scores. The MSP-SE dominance scores were used for comparative purposes with qualitative data.

Interviews were based on a semi-structured format and included open-ended questions; time restrictions limited the number of questions asked. The questions addressed participants' exercise behaviour, motivation for exercise, experience of possible withdrawal symptoms and perceptions of exercise dependence. Also included were questions relating to other characteristics of exercise dependence, such as engaging in exercise when injured or ill. Prior to the interviews, the interviewees were advised that the focus of the interview was exercise dependence. As a result, other topics such as eating disorders, anxiety conditions or personal circumstances were broached only when the participant invited discussion. The tape-recorded interviews were transcribed and coded using reversal theory concepts to identify motivational characteristics and participants' metamotivational processes in relation to exercise. Three judges, well versed in reversal theory, examined the coding independently and discussed any disagreements until consensus was reached.

Three of these short interview transcripts have been selected to illustrate the contrast in the responses of the individual exercisers, one categorized as primary and two exhibiting different kinds of secondary exercise dependence (see Figures 7.1, 7.2 and 7.3). MSP-SE dominance scores for the three exercisers are shown in Tables 7.2 and 7.3.

'Jim': primary exercise dependence

Jim, a 45-year-old male, scored 137 on the EDQ and 5 on the EAT measure, placing him firmly in the primary exercise dependent category. He showed a healthy BMI score, and there was no indication from the interview that he was overly concerned with weight or diet. Jim's exercise routine consisted of a daily run, which added up to an average of ten hours a week, and he often competed in cross-country events and marathon races as well. He was a runner who enjoyed achieving set goals within a strict training regime that also involved regular competition. He kept details of all his running logged in a training diary that he kept up to date religiously. Jim ran most days, scheduling his exercise around work and preferred to run early in the morning.

Jim liked his work as an aircraft engineer and felt that his exercise did not interfere with it. At the same time, he pointed out that he would never allow his job to interfere with his need to work out. He expressed the need to exercise in order to feel happy and said: 'Nothing I do replaces the feeling exercise gives me.' He felt that he was sensible in his approach to exercise and was able to cut back when sick or injured, although he also experienced feeling fed up, angry, bored or depressed when prevented from exercising (a finding also reported in Cox and Orford, 2004), but Jim's social life was not disrupted by his exercise activities.

The importance of his goal-setting and the enjoyment and gratification that he obtained from achieving them, along with his carefully planned running routine, reflect telic-oriented motivation that is typical of exercise dependent individuals. Jim's MSP-SE telic, autic and mastery dominance scores (see Table 7.2) are much higher than the average for the primary exercise dependence group and the highly active amateur sample as a whole. Jim appears to be a man very much in charge of his well-organized life and his responses to interview questions reflected his strong telic-autic-mastery personality.

'Clare': secondary exercise dependence (exercise dependence secondary to an eating disorder)

Clare, a 20-year-old female, scored 145 on the EDQ, 94 on the EAT instrument and had a BMI of 21.8. She was a registered eating disorder patient who also claimed to be dependent on exercise, averaging up to 20 hours every week. She was therefore classified as eating disordered with a secondary exercise dependence. She was very concerned about her weight and body image and felt that she was being controlled by her eating disorder. This

What is your exercise routine?
I run every day. Most mornings up to an hour and if I can't get my run in first thing I make sure I do it later in the day. I have over 32,000 miles of running logged in my training diary that I religiously keep up to date so I know that I am progressing and achieving my goals. I average about 10 hours of exercise a week and I run cross country and marathon competitions.
Do you work, what is your job?
I am an aircraft engineer.
How do your exercise sessions fit around your work?
I am an early riser and so run most mornings before work. I often go for longer runs at the weekend. I like getting up in the morning, as I feel so much better for it. It really sets me up for the day and I feel more alert and focused after my morning runs.
What is more important, your job or exercise?
I like both; they don't interfere, if anything they work well together. I run to make me feel good and stay fit and that in turn makes me more efficient and focused at work. I would never allow my job to interfere with my need to work out. So I could say my exercise is more important or comes first and foremost.
Would you miss work or other engagement in order to exercise?
I begrudge having to miss my weekend runs but I usually get a run in no matter what. Unless the weather is really bad I rarely miss a morning and during the winter I may adapt my workout to the gym. I would miss a workout if I had to but I couldn't take too much time off.
What is your goal for so much exercise or what do you hope to achieve?
I want to improve my marathon time and stay at a level of fitness where I enjoy running. I don't ever want to get to the point where I am struggling to run because I am unfit.
Do you ever cut your exercise session short when you feel tired or not well?
I will adapt my workout if I am sick. Sometimes there is no point in pushing yourself. I think I am fairly sensible but I struggle again to take too much time off.
How do you feel if you miss an exercise session?
Really fed up, angry. I was injured once and got really depressed. I find it hard to relax and get bored very quickly. I felt really frustrated and that I couldn't do the things I wanted to do. I felt I was being punished. I lost the identity running gives me and hated the way I looked and felt. Nothing I do replaces the feeling exercise gives me.
Do you feel you exercise enough? If you could would you do more?
Yes, I like the amount I do and can even feel OK about cutting it down but I could never stop. I always work hard for the up and coming race season. Although I am not very talented I consider myself an athlete and like to think I train like one.
Do you feel you have a problem?
I wouldn't call it a problem but I have a need and desire to exercise. Without it I am not happy.
What do your family and friends think of your exercise routine?
There is no problem really. I guess they are used to me. I fit my runs in wherever I can so it doesn't interfere too much.
Do you feel the same way about anything else in your life?
Not really but I am very passionate about most things I do, especially running. I guess I approach my life in a positive way; exercise really helps that.

Figure 7.1 'Jim': primary exercise dependence (from Blaydon, 2001)

What is your exercise routine?
I walk about 4-6 miles every day before work. I get up before work and do the same route. I also go to the gym and do aerobics classes in the evening and lunchtime.
Even when it is raining?
If it is bad I go to the gym and walk on the machine. I don't like doing that though but, I have to do something before I go to work it makes me feel good. I also swim three times a week in the evening.
Do you work, what is your job?
I work as a secretary and office administrator.
What are your hours?
I have to be in work by 9am and usually finish about 5 or 5.30pm.
What is more important, your job or exercise?
Definitely exercise. I don't like my job much, but I need the money
Would you miss work or other engagement in order to exercise?
Definitely, I don't go out much because I can't really cope with it. My problem is more my eating disorder, I don't mind going out for a drink but I won't go out for a meal.
Do you cook all your own food?
I have to be in control of my diet. As long as I know what I am eating I am ok. I have to have the same things then I am fine and I eat quite well. I have difficulty going out for a meal. I just think I am going to get fat. I have to prepare all my own food, I take my lunch into work, I never go out to lunch. I actually love cooking but I have such a fear of getting fat.
What is your goal for so much exercise or what do you hope to achieve?
I feel it controls my weight and keeps me healthy and fit looking. As long as I exercise I can eat. I hate it when I don't get my workout in. I feel so fat.
Do you ever cut your exercise session short when you feel tired or not well?
No never, I go crazy and I end up not eating. I think it is better to exercise and feel comfortable about yourself, than not eating.
Do you see any one about your eating problem?
I go to a local clinic and chat to them when I go through a really bad patch. I know I have a problem. It started when I left school and went to college. I thought I wasn't good enough to be there so I had to work really hard. I hated getting bad marks. It seemed that no matter how hard I tried I never got the top grades. I always felt so stupid. I have been told that my weight was one thing I could control and manipulate. Losing weight was the one thing I was good at. All the girls at school used to envy my body and ask how I stayed so slim. I felt I always looked the best and I like the attention I got from the boys. Unfortunately, it really developed into a problem and I started not eating or going out to dinner. I would eat an apple a day and a small dinner at night.
Do you still exercise if you are injured or ill?
I exercise no matter how I feel. It really makes me feel better. I can't not do it.
How do you feel if you miss an exercise session?
I get really depressed generally. Especially if I am having 'a fat day'. If I can't exercise on those days in particular, I feel really depressed. I exercise really hard if I have eaten something I feel I shouldn't. I am trying to get better but it is hard to break a habit I have had for so long. I like to keep calm and in control, especially around my food. Things start to go wrong when I can't control my life. I start to binge eat and exercise more to keep in control of my weight.
How do you feel after going out for a meal or made to eat something?
Meal times are so painful for me. I worry so much and get really nervous and angry inside. I get angry with everyone else as I think they are trying to make me fat so I find it easy then to just stop eating. I get really rebellious. I am learning to get better and my family has learnt to leave me alone but if someone says something to me I get really angry.
Do you feel you exercise enough. If you could would you do more?
I would do more if I could but I don't have the energy. Again, if I keep to my routine I am fine but if I break the routine I have to do more exercise to work off the extra calories.
What do your family and friends think of your exercise routine?
They really support me now but I don't think they really understand that this is a disease. I really want to get better and they have stood by me. I don't have many friends anymore. I don't go out anymore so they have stopped phoning me and I don't think they understand my problem. I think they think I am really sick. I hate that I have become like this, I am really embarrassed when I see my friends because I don't want them to know I am ill. I like the way I was so I spend a lot of time on my own.
Do you feel the same way about anything else in your life?
Not really, being thin is the most important thing in my life. I do hate that, I want to be normal again. I have put my family through so much, I feel so lonely and unhappy and I desperately want to get better.
Describe your personality for me.
I think I am a perfectionist. I am really tidy and I am really particular about my image especially my body image. I have become very shy and I used to be very outgoing but I am not anymore. I hate that this eating disorder controls my life.

Figure 7.2 'Clare': secondary exercise dependence (exercise dependence secondary to eating disorder) (from Blaydon, 2001)

What is your exercise routine?
I compete in triathlons. I run, bike and swim.
How much?
Anything from10 to 20 hours a week, depending on my goal. If I do Iron-man I train about 18-20 hours a week. I take one rest day a week, I am ok with that and I never miss a session.
Have you always competed in Triathlon?
No, I was a rugby player before. I played for a woman's team in the UK and then at national level for triathlon. I moved over to triathlon because I hated the politics behind the rugby here. I wasn't doing as well as I thought I should.
Why triathlon, is it so different?
I wanted to lose some weight and get fit. So I entered into a small run/swim race and won and that was me hooked, I thought this was relatively easy to do well in. I am fiercely competitive and success is really important to me.
How well do you do now?
I am getting better and better with time. It does take time for your body to adapt to the sport but I am a very determined person and quitting is just not an option for me. With hard work and determination and belief in myself I now race at a reasonable level. I will never be at the top but I think I can do better.
Do you think you are addicted to exercise?
Totally, I love the way it makes me feel, but the sport of triathlon has completely changed my life. When I played rugby I still drank and smoked. Now, I don't do either and I am obsessive about my food quality. I only put healthy stuff into my body so that I know I will have the energy to train.
Do you work; what is your job?
Unfortunately, I work in a bank looking after the computer systems. I work an average of 9-10 hours a day, sometimes more.
How do your exercise sessions fit around your work?
I work out in the morning before work everyday, I work out at lunch and some evenings. The weekends are taken up with racing or training that I leave for my long sessions. I train in the morning because by the evening I am too tired. I find it hard to motivate myself. I have to go straight to a swim session because if I go home I will not train.
What is more important, your job or exercise?
Definitely exercise. Unfortunately, I can't afford to do triathlon without work. Work pays for my trips and equipment so I guess I work so that I can do triathlon to the level that I do. I quite like work really, it is different and a break from my routine.
Would you miss work or other engagements in order to exercise?
I never miss a work out and I will not go to the engagement without working out before hand if I have to. I will let people know if I am going to be late. If I am training and the engagement clashes, I will work out instead. If I have breakfast meetings at work I just get up earlier and work out then.
What is your goal for so much exercise or what do you hope to achieve?
I want to be a better triathlete. I also want to continue enjoying the sport. I also want to look like

Figure 7.3 'Bev': secondary exercise dependence (eating disorder secondary to exercise dependence) (from Blaydon, 2001)

appeared to be a constant battle and a focus of anxiety in her life. Clare's need for control was tied up with her need to keep calm. For example, when her eating routine was upset she would begin to feel anxious and would turn to exercise to retrieve a sense of control over her body. The importance of having control in her life is typical of secondary exercise dependent individuals and others with eating disorders (it also seems to be important to some primary exercise dependent individuals as seen in Cox and Orford's (2004) *exercising control* category). Like Jim, Clare also became depressed and irritable when forced to abstain from exercise, especially on one of her 'fat' days. However, exercise helped Clare to feel good (a point also reported by quite an athlete. I am very competitive and so would like to be faster than the other triathletes here in Hong Kong. I also want to beat my personal best and I guess I have dreams of being really successful but I am happy with what I am achieving now. I always have small goals and I always achieve them. I just work harder to get there if they are tough goals. I hate to fail.

Do you ever cut your exercise session short when you feel tired or not well?

I have done, but it is rare. If I am going to work out for 47 minutes I will work out for 47 minutes. I am getting better though. I am beginning to listen to my body and understand it. If it is tired I will ease back a bit but I won't miss a session.

Do you still exercise if you are injured or ill?

It depends, I haven't had a bad injury. If I am very sick I do try and rest but I find it hard. I have to be very sick. I do tend to train if I only have a cold, things like that don't really affect me.

How do you feel if you miss an exercise session?

Awful, I get really angry with myself if I have to miss sessions. I can't bear it so I don't. I just can't settle down and I think I am going to get fat and unfit. I really try not to miss a session. I have to travel with work and I enjoy that but if I am training for a race I will take my bike so that I can train.

Do you feel you exercise enough? If you could would you do more?

I used to think that I could do more. Through experience I have learned what my body can cope with and what it can't. I used to be able to only manage 10 hours a week and feel bad as everyone else was doing 18. So I tried and I couldn't cope; I got pretty tired. I have managed, subconsciously, to push my hours higher and longer as I have got fitter. I can now do these big hours but I would only do it every now and again if I am aiming for an Iron-man. If I didn't have to work then I would do more. I would always do a base of 10 hours to maintain my fitness. It is my routine now, I have to do what I have said I would.

Do you feel you have a problem?

Not really, I used to smoke and drink and eat really badly so I don't feel that bad. I like what I do and I like my life. I don't care if other people think I am crazy. I love exercise and I love the way it makes me feel. It is that feeling that gets me up in the morning.

What do your family and friends think of your exercise routine?

They think I am mad. Most of my friends compete but I guess I do train more. I am pretty competitive and it makes me feel better if I do more. I think everyone including other triathletes think I am crazy getting up at 4.30am for a three hour work out before work but I have to do it, I need to be in control of my routine and know I am working hard. I guess I am pretty bossy at work too. I get really angry if I don't get things done or if other people are lazy. I guess people have got used to me and my ways. I don't care about what others think anyway, I do what I want to do.

Do you feel the same way about anything else in your life?

I put 100 per cent into everything; there is no point doing it otherwise, but I guess triathlon is my most important. I always need to be achieving whether at work or sport

Describe your personality for me

Focused, single minded, determined, selfish, stubborn, planner and committed/disciplined. Can be a perfectionist and a bit obsessive.

Table 7.2 MSP-SE dominance scores for 'Jim' – primary exercise dependence (from Blaydon, 2001)

| | MSP-SE scores | |
	'Jim'(Primary)	*Primary group mean*
Telic	10	2
Arousal avoidance	3	−2
Negativism	− 8	−6
Autic	11	1
Mastery	6	−1
Optimism	7	9

* scores rounded to nearest integer

Table 7.3 MSP-SE scores for secondary exercise dependent interviewees 'Clare'
(exercise dependence secondary to eating disorder) and 'Bev' (eating
disorder secondary to exercise dependence) (from Blaydon, 2001)

| | MSP-SE scores | | |
	'Clare' (ex sec to eat)	'Bev' (eat sec to ex)	Secondary group mean
Telic	10	14	11
Arousal avoidance	14	8	7
Negativism	−15	− 6	−10
Autic	− 3	9	− 1
Mastery	− 2	6	0
Optimism	−11	−20	− 6

* scores rounded to nearest integer

a few of the interviewees in the Bamber *et al.* (2000b, 2003) study). Her
eating problems and exercise activities had badly affected her social life.
This might be partly due to the fact that she thought of herself as a
perfectionist who used to be outgoing, but had become very shy. All of this
tied in with her strongly pessimistic outlook as shown by her highly negative
score on MSP-SE optimism dominance (see Table 7.3).

Clare's description of her feelings and attitudes are in accord with her
much higher than average scores on MSP-SE arousal avoidance dominance
and much lower than average score on negativism. Clare is very conformist,
as evidenced by the way that she coped with her eating disorder by keeping
in control of her diet and being very careful about eating the same things.
With the importance of self-control, Clare might have been expected to
have relatively high MSP-SE autic and mastery dominance scores. However,
as can be seen from Table 7.3, these exercise context dominance scores for
Clare and her group are low and negative, indicating that these secondary
exercise dependent exercisers are slightly alloic and sympathy dominant.
Why this should be is not apparent. Being highly arousal avoidant, Clare
pointed out in her interview that family meal times could be highly
threatening situations for her and sometimes she became angry and rebelled
by refusing to eat.

**'Bev': secondary exercise dependence (eating disorder secondary
to exercise dependence)**

Bev, a 27-year-old female, scored 149 on the EDQ, 72 on the EAT and had
a BMI of just 18.1. Although she could be classified as secondary exercise
dependent based on these scores, it was not entirely clear from the interview
how prevalent her eating disorder was, as she clearly explained that the

focus of her exercise and concern with weight was performance related. Her eating problem was secondary to her exercise dependence. She was concerned about only eating quality food so that she had the energy to train and described a fear of getting fat if she did not exercise. She also wanted to look like an athlete and so was also concerned about her body image.

Bev competed in Ironman triathlons and many smaller events where she had reached a high level of competition. She often completed 20 hours of exercise activities per week, which she had to fit in around a full-time job. She said that she was a perfectionist and was clearly very determined and focused in her competitiveness and the highly structured pattern of her training (e.g. getting up at 4.30 a.m. for a three-hour workout before work), which left her little time for social life.

She also described the many positive benefits she experienced from her sport and exercise and enjoyed both physical and emotional rewards. It was also evident that her lifestyle habits had drastically changed since taking up triathlon and these appeared to have had a positive effect on her health and performance. These positive changes in health and performance appeared to justify and reinforce her excessive exercise behaviour. For example, she also made it clear that she would never miss a training session because of worry about gaining weight and losing fitness if she missed too much (see Chapter 5).

The descriptions of Bev's very intensive exercise and competition activities fit neatly with her telic, autic and mastery MSP-SE dominance scores. Her scores were all higher than average for the secondary exercise dependent group and much higher than the average for the whole sample of highly active amateurs, but typical for the highly competitive amateur triathletes (Blaydon et al., 2002). Her high MSP-SE pessimism score corresponds well with her low expectations of future success in the triathlon as expressed in the interview (see Table 7.3).

The four qualitative studies compared

Although the four studies used different approaches to analysing and interpreting the qualitative data that was obtained in interviews with intensive exercisers, definitive profiles of secondary and primary exercisers have begun to emerge. When the quotations presented in the different studies are examined, a good deal of common ground and even overlap can be seen in the experiences of dependent exercisers.

For example, interviews yielded a good deal of information about secondary exercise dependent exercisers (Bamber et al., 2000b, 2003; Blaydon, 2001; Yates, 1991). Virtually all these exercisers showed a need for control of their bodies and were very concerned about weight, diet and body shape. The majority had clinical eating disorders or problematic eating behaviour. For some of the interviewees, exercise was secondary to an eating disorder; for others the eating disorder was secondary to the exercise. Exercise was the central feature of their lives, to the extent that it impaired their psychological, social and occupational, physical and behavioural functioning. Many were fearful of not being able to exercise, continued to exercise when sick or injured and experienced withdrawal symptoms when prevented from exercising. Some of these exercisers tried to conceal the amount of exercise that they did. However, for many, exercise made them feel better, and they used it to modulate mood when feeling anxious or depressed, with the added benefit that it led to improved self-esteem and self-confidence.

In the case of primary exercise dependence, Bamber et al. (2003) proposed that the new criteria that they developed for secondary exercise dependence might also be used to identify primary exercise dependence where there was no evidence of an eating disorder. Material from interviews with exercisers in the Blaydon (2001) and Cox and Orford (2004) studies tended to support this proposal, as a number of similar features of exercise behaviour were found in primary exercise dependent interviewees. By way of illustration, exercising control and creating a pleasing body shape (generally without the accompanying intense focus on weight and diet found in secondary dependent exercisers) were also found with these interviewees. Exercise was of major importance to these interviewees, and they too used exercise to regulate mood for short-term psychological benefits and longer-term improvements in self-confidence and general well being. Quite a number of them were also fearful of not being able to exercise, exercised when ill or injured, and experienced negative mood when unable to do so.

These four studies have produced some rich and detailed descriptive data about the experience of those involved in highly intensive exercise. They have made a useful contribution to the literature on exercise dependence and provided enhanced insights into the psychological processes involved.

Closing comments

Each of the studies reviewed in this chapter utilized a qualitative approach to data gathering, and three of them also used quantitative measures to identify the various participants to be interviewed. This combined approach is a potentially powerful research strategy that unfortunately was only partially successful. Some of the problems in identifying primary exercise dependence were associated with the EDQ and choice of cut-off point for exercise dependence. The validity of the EDQ as a measure of dependence was actually questioned by Cox and Orford (2004) as it was originally only validated against a measure of eating disorders (EAT) and a measure of mood (Profile of Mood States, POMS; McNair, Lorr and Droppleman, 1985), but not against another measure of dependence. Ogden et al.'s. (1997) EDQ was the first scale developed to measure symptoms of exercise dependence, but, as Bamber et al. (2003) pointed out, diagnosis should involve clinical psychology interview procedures as the EDQ is not a diagnostic instrument. The more recently developed and more rigorously validated Exercise Dependence

Scale (EDS; Hausenblas and Symons Downs, 2002) may prove to be a more sensitive scale than the EDQ and could, therefore, prove useful in future research.

Cox and Orford's category, *scratching an itch or setting a goal*, is a particularly interesting finding for the context of this book for two reasons. First, Brown (1997) underlined the importance of planning in the management of good hedonic tone in his Hedonic Management Model of Addiction, and the long-term aims and goals of the Cox and Orford (2004) interviewees may merely be a way of ensuring that their regular short-term psychological pay-offs would remain accessible. Second, this category, as described by the authors in the quote earlier in the present chapter (Cox and Orford, 2004, p. 184) epitomizes the reversal theory concept of the relationship between the telic and paratelic pair of metamotivational states and the reversals that occur between them. Within reversal theory it is perfectly possible for the pleasures of the short-term buzz to be juxtaposed with the achievement of long-term performance goals. The former is characteristic of a paratelic (playful, spontaneous, present-oriented, non-goal oriented) and the latter of a telic (serious, goal oriented, forward planning) orientation to exercise. It is possible for different people to experience these different orientations, and for the same person to experience both these orientations at different times. Neither *scratching the itch* nor *setting the goal* was considered exclusive by the researchers in this sample of high frequency exercisers. There is a relationship between them that Brown's (1997) model and reversal theory can help to explain.

According to Cox and Orford (2004), evidence supporting an addiction framework came from the *price to pay* category in terms of the negative consequences of engaging in long-term intensive exercise (e.g. exercising when ill or injured and sometimes against medical advice). These negative consequences of intensive activity are important elements in Brown's (1997) model, as are the short-term pay-offs in mood and long-term improvements in hedonic tone found in Cox and Orford's (2004) study. The authors also pointed out that some of their other results did not fit into an addiction framework, such as a focus on long-term goals concerning health or body shape. However, these can also be explained by Brown's (1997) model, which underlined the importance of planning in the management of good hedonic tone. The long-term health goals of Cox and Orford's (2004) interviewees may merely be a way of ensuring that their regular short-term psychological boosts in hedonic tone would remain ongoing as they progressed towards their long-term exercise goals. In similar fashion to long-term health goals, exercisers might undertake long-term planning with regard to their body shape, knowing that the periodic achievements that they observe through measurement (e.g. increases in muscle size) have the potential to boost hedonic tone through the transactional emotions and feelings of satisfaction and pride as they take steps along the road to achieving their ideal body shape.

Finally, several of the negative aspects of secondary exercise dependence (e.g. impaired functioning, withdrawal and denial) found in the interviews (Bamber *et al.*, 2000b, 2003; Blaydon, 2001; Yates, 1991) also fit Brown's (1997) model of addiction.

References

American Psychiatric Association (1994) *Diagnostic and statistical manual of mental disorders* (4th edition), Washington DC: American Psychiatric Association.

Apter, M. J., Mallows, R. and Williams, S. (1998) 'The development of the Motivational Style Profile', *Personality and Individual Differences*, 24, 7–18.

Bamber, D., Cockerill, I. M. and Carroll, D. (2000a) 'The pathological status of exercise dependence', *British Journal of Sports Medicine*, 34, 125–32.

Bamber, D., Cockerill, I. M., Rodgers, S. and Carroll, D. (2000b) '"It's exercise or nothing": A qualitative analysis of exercise dependence', *British Journal of Sports Medicine*, 34, 423–30.

Bamber, D., Cockerill, I. M., Rodgers, S. and Carroll, D. (2003) 'Diagnostic criteria for exercise dependence in women', *British Journal of Sports Medicine*, 37, 393–400.

Blaydon, M. J. (2001) *Descriptive and metamotivational characteristics of primary and secondary exercise dependent and eating disordered participants in intense physical activity*, unpublished doctoral dissertation, Hong Kong: The University of Hong Kong.

Blaydon, M. J., Lindner, K. J. and Kerr, J. H. (2002) 'Metamotivational characteristics of eating-disordered and exercise-dependent triathletes', *Psychology of Sport and Exercise*, 3, 223–36.

Blaydon, M. J., Lindner, K. J. and Kerr, J. H. (2004) 'Metamotivational characteristics of exercise dependence and eating disorders in highly active amateur sport participants', *Personality and Individual Differences*, 36, 1419–32.

Brown, R. I. F. (1997) 'A theoretical model of behavioural addictions – Applied to offending', in J. E. Hodge, M. McMurran and C. R. Hollin (eds) *Addicted to crime?*, New York: Wiley, 13–65.

Charmaz, K. (1990) 'Discovering chronic illness: Using grounded theory', *Sociology of Science and Medicine*, 30, 1161–72.

Charmaz, K. (1995) 'Grounded theory', in J. A. Smith, R. Harre and L. Langenhove (eds) *Rethinking methods in psychology*, London: Sage.

Cox, R. and Orford, J. (2004) 'A qualitative study of the meaning of exercise for people who could be labelled as "addicted" to exercise – Can "addiction" be applied to high frequency exercising?, *Addiction Research and Theory*, 12, 167–88.

Fairburn, C. G. and Beglin, S. J. (1994) 'Assessment of eating disorders: interview or self-report questionnaire?', *International Journal of Eating Disorders*, 16, 363–70.

Fairburn, C. G. and Cooper, Z. (1993) 'The Eating Disorder Examination', in C. G. Fairburn and G. T. Wilson (eds) *Binge eating: Nature, assessment and treatment*, New York: Guildford Press.

Garner, D. M. and Garfinkel, P. E. (1979) 'The Eating Attitudes Test: An index of the symptoms of anorexia nervosa', *Psychological Medicine*, 9, 273–9.

Glaser, B. and Strauss, A. (1967) *The discovery of grounded theory*, Chicago IL: Aldine.

Hausenblas, H. A. and Symons Downs, D. (2002) 'How much is too much? The development and validation of the Exercise Dependence Scale', *Psychology and Health*, 17, 387–404.

Henwood, K. L. (1996) 'Qualitative inquiry: Perspectives, methods, and psychology', in J. T. E. Richardson (ed.) *Handbook of qualitative research methods for psychology and the social sciences*, Leicester: The British Psychological Society.

McNair, D. M., Lorr, M. and Droppleman, L. F. (1985) *The Profile of Mood States manual*, San Diego CA: Educational and Industrial Testing Services.

Ogden, J., Veale, D. M. W. and Summers, Z. (1997) 'The development and validation of the Exercise Dependence Questionnaire', *Addiction Research*, 5, 343–56.

Orford, J. (2001) *Excessive appetites: A psychological view of addictions*, Chichester: John Wiley.

QSR NUD*IST 4.0 (1993) *User guide*, London: Sage.

Strauss, A. and Corbin, J. (1990) *Basics of qualitative research: Grounded theory procedures and techniques*, Sage: London.

Szabo, A. (2000) 'Physical activity as a source of psychological dysfunction', in S. J. H. Biddle, K. R. Fox and S. H. Boutcher (eds) *Physical activity and psychological well-being*, London: Routledge, 130–95.

Veale, D. (1995) 'Does primary exercise dependence really exist?', in J. Annett, B. Cripps and H. Steinberg (eds) *Exercise addiction: Motivation for participation in sport and exercise*, Leicester: The British Psychological Society, 1–5.

Yates, A. (1991) *Compulsive exercise and the eating disorders*, New York: Brunner Mazel.

Yates, A., Leehey, K. and Shisslak, C. M. (1983) 'Running: An analogue of anorexia?', *New England Journal of Medicine*, 308, 251–5.

8 Taking stock
Return to Brown's (1997) model and possible intervention

This chapter will examine primary exercise dependence in the light of Brown's (1997) Hedonic Management Model of Addictions and reversal theory (e.g. Apter, 2001) extensions to the model. It will be argued that primary exercise dependence does exist as a separate entity and that it is a true pathological condition. Finally, some strategies for assisting people with primary and secondary exercise dependence will be proposed.

The evidence presented throughout this book has been quite conclusive about the pathological nature of secondary exercise dependence, both where the exercise is secondary to an eating disorder and where the eating disorder is secondary to exercise dependence. For the former, this evidence has ranged from the recognition by clinical psychologists that some of their clients presenting with eating disorders were also engaged in excessive exercise behaviour (e.g. Long et al., 1993; Veale, 1995) to the results of research studies that included secondary exercise dependent participants (e.g. Bamber et al., 2000a, 2000b, 2003; Blaydon, 2001; Blaydon et al., 2002, 2004; Yates, 1991). For the latter, interview material and the results of research studies on, for example, elite athletes with eating disorders participating in endurance sports have also supported this conclusion (see Chapter 5; e.g. Downes, 1998; Hulley and Hill, 2001; Sundgot-Borgen, 1993, 1994a, 1994b). The attitudes, motivation and excessive exercising behaviour of these secondary exercise dependent individuals fit well with Brown's (1997) Hedonic Management Model of Addictions and substantiate the pathological nature of both types of the condition.

In Chapter 1, attention was drawn to some observers who have raised questions about whether primary exercise dependence actually exists and whether it is a real pathology (e.g. Keski-Rahkonen, 2001; Veale, 1995). Now, as the end of this book is approached, it is appropriate to ask if it is possible to reach more definite conclusions about the existence and pathological nature of primary exercise dependence. In order to adjudicate on this issue, a re-examination of some of the available evidence in the light of Brown's (1997) model might prove helpful. If it can be shown that the attitudes, motivation and ensuing behaviour of so-called primary exercise dependent individuals are in close accord with the first seven propositions of Brown's (1997) model, there should be little doubt that primary exercise dependence is an addiction and the condition is pathological.

Brown's (1997) model and primary exercise dependence

The first seven propositions or stages of Brown's (1997) model are: (1) management of hedonic tone; (2) vulnerabilities; (3) initiation; (4) addictive activity choice; (5) development of an acquired drive and increasing salience; (6) cycles; and (7) established addiction. Each of these will be summarized and examined below in relation to the available evidence on primary exercise dependence.

Management of hedonic tone

Individuals learn to maintain good hedonic tone by manipulating their arousal levels, mood and experience of their own feelings of well-being. This allows them to maintain pleasant mental states and feelings of general happiness for long periods. If, for example, individuals find that exercise activities can be used to bring about increases or decreases in felt arousal, manipulating arousal through exercise may become a central element in how they manage their hedonic tone. The results of empirical studies reported in Chapter 3 support this notion. Results have indicated that exercise can bring about increases in arousal (Kerr and Vlaswinkel, 1993; Kerr and van den Wollenberg, 1997), as well as increases in pleasant, and decreases in unpleasant, emotions (Kerr and Kuk, 2001). It was also shown that exercise can have a tension-reducing function (Thayer *et al.*, 1994) and an anxiety-reducing function (Biddle and Mutrie, 2001). Further, Thayer *et al.* (1994) demonstrated that exercise was the most effective behavioural category for changing a bad mood. Research evidence from these studies (and other evidence presented in this book, for example, interview transcripts) shows that it is certainly possible that a person who experiments with exercise may well discover that it can be used in the self-regulation of mood and arousal to produce positive hedonic tone. For some individuals, this may be the first step on the way to primary exercise dependence.

Vulnerabilities

Some people may have predispositions that make them vulnerable to addictions by increasing the size of the individual's hedonic gap (difference between the level of negative feeling states a person can tolerate and the level they experience), and reducing the number of easily accessible rewarding activities available to them. One of the vulnerabilities identified by Brown is individual differences in personality and temperament: Brown argued that those with a personality that was oriented to sensation seeking (as measured by the Sensation Seeking Scale; SSS; Zuckerman, 1979) were more likely to become addicted to 'experience changing substances and experiences' than those who were not sensation-seekers.

The results of the Hong Kong studies reviewed in Chapter 6 appear to contradict this for dependent exercisers. For example, in Blaydon *et al.*'s (2002) study of triathletes, the Motivational Style Profile (MSP: Apter *et al.*, 1998) results showed that the primary exercise dependent triathletes' scores on the arousal-avoidance dimension were significantly higher than those of the control group. (The MSP arousal-seeking and arousal-avoidance subscale is closely related to SSS sensation seeking; see Trimpop *et al.*, 1999.) This finding points to dependent exercisers having personalities that are arousal avoidant rather than arousal seeking. However, the hedonic gap works both ways in addictions. Sensation seeking addicts will choose activities that reduce the hedonic gap by increasing arousal to obtain excitement (e.g. gamblers). Other addicts obtain calm and control by closing their hedonic gap through decreasing arousal (e.g. by taking certain drugs or exercising). Consequently, Brown's argument can be extended to include personality types that might be vulnerable to addictions because they are arousal avoidant (e.g. primary exercise dependent exercisers) and seek to reduce arousal levels.

Initiation

The individual finds an activity that can act as a powerful means of manipulating, and maintaining extended periods of positive hedonic tone through gradual realization or sudden discovery. This activity then takes priority over other easily accessible rewarding activities. There is ample evidence in the sources referred to in this book of the power of exercise to bring about positive changes to mood and its potential to become an important aspect of some people's lives. Individuals who initially undertake exercise in small doses, running around the block or taking the dog for a walk, may find that they enjoy it and progress on to longer distances and more frequent exercising. For example, in a study of women attending a city health and fitness club, two highly intensive exercisers described how they began and how their attendance escalated:

> Someone came into the office and offered a complimentary visit. I now come to escape from my sedentary job, and I find I manage to wind down through exercise.
>
> Exercise tends to be an addictive thing. You start off by going a couple of times a week and end up going every day. If I don't go at least four times a week my mind and body don't feel the benefits.
>
> (Redican and Hadley, 1988, pp. 56, 58)

Other dependent exercisers' initiation is more sudden and extreme. One 25-year-old man (who later developed eating problems at college), spoke about his initiation to running in high school and how he came to enjoy it: 'I immediately joined in the 10-mile daily workout and was expected to run no less than 70 miles a week. This was a challenge at first, but very soon I began to relish it' (Yates, 1991, p. 26).

Addictive activity choice

Brown identified four important factors in an individual's choice of additive activity, including the range of activities available to the individual, whether there was social support for the activity, the effectiveness of the inherent properties of the activity to affect hedonic tone (especially those that are reinforcing), and the skills the individual has acquired for manipulating hedonic tone. Exercise is both easily accessible and is viewed as socially acceptable, and its effect on hedonic tone is evident from interview material, as illustrated by these two quotes from Cathy:

> I got a buzz from the other stuff, from running and swimming, I got a buzz because it makes you feel so good . . . there's that . . . what I call a 'sweet' moment when everything comes together, when you get everything right when you're doing your sport . . . and it feels great.

> I think part of a distinction is health . . . I suppose to a certain extent society's views because to exercise is healthy and to exercise is good, to take drugs is unhealthy so it's socially unacceptable so I suppose that plays some part in it as well.
>
> (Cox and Orford, 2004, p. 181)

Cathy's comments not only illustrate the potential that exercise has for becoming an addiction, but also show how intensive exercise is often seen by others as a 'positive' addiction that is acceptable and preferable to alternative unhealthy addictions. This general attitude to exercise provides the primary exercise dependent exerciser with the social support that Brown has pointed out was important in this fourth stage of his model.

Development of an acquired drive and increasing salience

Once a person's goal to achieve specific mood states becomes an acquired drive and a single activity takes on increasing importance as a source of reward, the person concerned is liable to develop an addiction. A cycle is set up where increases in the salience of the single activity bring about increases in tolerance, withdrawals and relief action, which lead to even greater salience. For some individuals, exercise can gradually become so important that it becomes a central feature of life and is often perceived as more important than any other activity, to the point that it can interfere with their work and/or their social interactions. As one primary exercise dependent exerciser commented when asked about the relationship between exercise and his work:

> Exercise is everything to me and definitely more important . . . Because there is generally no pattern to my work schedule this means I often have 'free' days. Otherwise, I exercise at lunchtime or when travelling to and from work. For example, in the summer I cycled to work most days and returned by train about 20 miles. Sometimes I run part of the way (8 miles) or on the odd occasion the full journey.
>
> (Blaydon, 2001, p. 116)

Others find themselves getting up early and putting in hours of exercise before work; many of these exercisers talk about feeling driven to continue exercising when ill or injured, often against medical advice (Blaydon, 2001; Cox and Orford, 2004). Rather than suffer the negative mood or withdrawal symptoms from not exercising, they are prepared to risk their health. Typical of this attitude is a quote from Andy who, when asked if he would stop when told to do so, said:

> No I'd adapt my exercise . . . I wouldn't reduce it but I may do other things . . . because I know what it's like not to exercise . . . I mean I pulled a muscle about two years ago and had two weeks off, the doctor said I should have had six . . . I had two weeks off and it was horrible. I wouldn't want to spend 30 years feeling like that, I probably wouldn't change cause they (medics) are full of s..t anyway.
>
> (Cox and Orford, 2004, p. 183)

When the attitudes and behaviour of primary exercise dependent individuals are examined, it is clear that, for many, the salience of exercise has become pre-eminent and their tolerance for exercise has increased to the point where they abhor the unpleasant withdrawal symptoms they experience when prevented from exercising, and must continue to exercise to relieve them.

Cycles

Classical conditioning and reinforcement schedules play a role in the development of repeated cycles that make up a serial of addictive activity. During these serials of addictive activity, the individual has developed rituals and routines that induce the desired mental states, and cognitive and belief systems may have become distorted and dysfunctional. For the addicted exerciser, doing without exercise is not an option and many appear to be quite skilled in adapting their daily exercise to fit in with the rest of their lives. This often involves self-imposed routines and structures that are strictly followed (Cox and Orford, 2004). One participant from Blaydon's (2001) study was a 49-year-old semi-retired consultant who spent three to four hours a day working out. (Although his EDQ score of 116 placed him in the no-dependence group in that study, it was similar to the scores of the exercise dependent participants in the 2004 Cox and Orford study.) He explained:

> I really tailor my life to fit around my exercise routine. Exercise has replaced the time I spent at work so I still socialize in the evenings. I wouldn't miss my exercise unless it was a real necessity . . . I am addicted. I don't think I have a problem but I love exercise and I hate the way I feel when I don't do my work out . . . My symptoms are most definitely both physical and emotional and I feel they are linked together. I don't have an eating disorder. I love my food.
>
> (Blaydon, 2001, pp. 139–40)

It is obvious that, to be heavily involved in exercise and to develop effective daily exercise routines, a degree of planning is required. Planning allows the dependent exerciser to use a reliable method to manipulate arousal levels in the desired direction, thus contributing to the effective management of hedonic tone over time (Brown, 1997). Strict adherence to the routines and structures that these exercisers build for themselves can be compared to the cycles and serials of addictive activity described by Brown in this stage of his model. The ritual of entering exercise facilities or setting out on favoured exercise routes induces the desired mental states. The regular experience of these states, along with each successful completion of exercise session goals and periodic improvements in fitness or physique, provides ongoing reinforcement for continuing exercise activity.

Established addiction

At this stage, feelings and behaviour are totally dominated by one particular addictive activity in a motivational monopoly. That activity is now the only source of reward in a person's life and crucial to maintaining positive mood, accompanied by increasing conflict and the continuous desire to avoid withdrawal. Joanna, the 25-year-old Jiu-Jitsu athlete, whose attitudes to exercise and excessive exercise behaviour were detailed in Griffiths' (1997) case study (see Chapter 2), provides the perfect example of an athlete who has progressed to stage seven of Brown's model and exhibits all the core components of someone who is addicted to exercise: 'There is no doubt (at least in the author's mind) that Joanna was (and probably still is) addicted to exercise and that she displays all the core components of any bona fide addiction' (Griffiths, 1997, p. 165).

Joanna, like the majority of the primary exercise dependent people encountered in the various research studies, recognized that her exercise was a problem, but did not consider herself addicted. Some of these exercisers did use the word 'addicted' when describing their attitude to exercise, but were quick to qualify it by adding that they were addicted, but 'not in a negative way like other addictions' (see Cathy's comments above). Joanna's attitude to exercise was similar to that expressed by Cox, the first author in the Cox and Orford (2004) study, in a personal statement. As a committed exerciser herself, she argued that: 'I certainly did not feel 'addicted' or that I was inflicting harm upon myself, I had never felt better, and yet this label could have been attached to me' (Cox and Orford, 2004, p. 174).

Cox's stance is not unique, but it does contrast with the view held by some of the participants in her own study. Henry, for example, was not convinced by the argument that exercise is healthy:

> I still think that there's this misconception that exercise is really healthy for us . . . I know I'm fit at the moment but I don't know how healthy I am . . . and as a competitive runner we are not doing twenty minutes three times a week as it is recommended we do . . . we are far over that so whereas we get fit I'm not sure that we are that healthy . . . I think that there is a price to pay somewhere along the line . . .
>
> (Cox and Orford, 2004, p. 183)

There is an old saying about gambling addiction: 'It's only a gambling problem if you are losing.' It may be that something similar holds for exercise dependence. In other words, being addicted to highly intensive exercise may not be problematic while everything is going well, but once prolonged exercise causes injury, or people continue to exercise when injured or ill (because exercise has become the only means of maintaining positive hedonic tone), exercise can be seen as being just as destructive as some other addictions. 'Losing' in the exercise context can also mean the negative effect that excessive exercise can have on family relations, social life and work. Addicted exercisers may not be so different from addicts who use alcohol to achieve psychological benefits and also pay the long-term price of damage to their bodies.

What has emerged from the research studies reviewed in Chapters 6 and 7 is primarily a profile of secondary exercise dependence. Given that the Bamber *et al.* (2003) study focused only on secondary exercise dependent exercisers, it may have been premature for them to suggest that their secondary exercise dependent criteria could be used for diagnosing primary exercise dependence. However, in the light of interview research results (e.g. Blaydon, 2001; Cox and Orford, 2004; Griffiths, 1997) it seems possible. In fact, many of the diagnostic criteria could also be applied to other dependencies, for example, alcohol or drugs (e.g. impaired functioning, withdrawal, conflict), and are also in accord with Brown's seventh proposition about what constitutes an established addiction.

Furthermore, if the statements that relate to food and diet are deleted, Yates' (1991) description of 'obligatory' runners could very easily serve as a description of the attitude, motivation and behaviour of primary exercise dependent exercisers:

Obligatory runners are individuals who know pain. They compromise their bodies by continuing to run when injured. They forfeit jobs, marriages, friends, and other pleasures because of their running regimen. They plan vacations around running and when they are not running they ruminate endlessly about time, distance, . . . and the proper shoes . . . They retire early in the evening and may begin running well before dawn. They almost always run alone. There is nothing in their lives that can equal the experience of running.

(Yates, 1991, p. 29)

From the discussion above it should now be evident that the characteristics of primary exercise dependence are consistent with Brown's (1997) seven propositions or stages in the development of addiction; Brown himself recognized that high frequency exercising could become an addiction, including it among the fundamental addictions. Therefore it seems clear that some high frequency exercisers can be classified as primary exercise dependent and suffer from a true pathological condition.

Brown extended his 1997 model with some additional explanations of the motivational processes involved in addictions using conceptual arguments from reversal theory (Apter, 1982, 2001; Brown, 1988, 2001). In this regard, the following section examines how reversal theory can be applied to the comments that exercise dependent exercisers have made and add to the understanding of exercise dependence.

Insights from reversal theory

One of the interesting features of the results of the qualitative studies on exercise dependence reviewed in Chapter 7 was the enthusiastic and detailed manner in which people talked about their attitudes and feelings towards exercise, as well as its effect on their physical and psychological health, social relationships and everyday living. Among the quotes attributed to the high frequency exercisers in the interview studies in Chapter 7 were several that illustrate different types of metamotivation related to the participants' exercise experience.

One secondary exercise dependent triathlete (Bev), highlighted in Chapter 7, described the satisfaction and pleasure she obtained from achieving her exercise goals. The quote indicates the serious, telic orientation of her motivation for exercise:

Training makes me feel good in the sense you can quantify the improvement and see the benefits of your work unlike many other things in life. It is easy to set goals and work towards achieving them, satisfying the hunger to perform and do well.

(Blaydon, 2001, p. 125)

Peta, a 40-year-old with a BMI of 16, who vomited up to 20 times a day and alternated between severely restricting her eating and bingeing, used exercise to enable her to have some control over her weight and body shape. Every day was totally structured around her need to exercise. As she stated:

> if I don't do anything I feel heavy and so I feel low and so I'm more tempted to nibble and then a nibble makes me feel guilty so it turns into a binge . . . (exercise) . . . can make me feel quite in control, make me feel quite powerful over my eating . . . that's the foremost thing in my life.
>
> (Bamber *et al.*, 2000b, p. 428)

This quote shows both the serious, compliant (telic-conformity) and self-focused control (autic-mastery) motives behind her exercising. Planning her life around exercise and conforming to and completing her regimen played an important role in the positive feelings she experienced as she controlled her weight and maintained her body shape. Not exercising changed her experience, invoking unpleasant feelings of negative hedonic tone (feeling low and 'heavy') and guilt (before a binge). Feeling sorry for herself when she felt 'low' (autic-sympathy) may have been what triggered the temptation to nibble and start off a binge.

Another secondary dependent exerciser (Jenny), who was forced to engage in vigorous walking because cycling 60–80 miles per day had resulted in a back problem, noted a severe adverse response to exercise withdrawal, including extreme anxiety, depression, lack of concentration and insomnia:

> I just feel tied up in a knot really . . . like really tense and agitated and erm [sic], as if I have had something taken away, that's how I feel, I feel really cross and annoyed and something has been taken away that I think is mine . . .
>
> (Bamber *et al.*, 2000b, p. 427)

When forced to reduce exercise activity, Jenny's feelings of tension and loss are indicative of low felt transactional outcome and possible loss of control (autic-mastery). The influence of the telic and negativistic states, reflected in her feelings of being 'cross and annoyed', as well as her feelings of anxiety, were also major contributors to the tension she experienced. Her resentment (autic-sympathy) at being unable to exercise indicates a probable reversal from the mastery to the sympathy state.

Motivational process involved in exercise addiction

In Chapter 3, it was pointed out that there were three likely reversal theory explanations of the motivational processes involved in exercise addiction:

arousal modulation, reversal inhibition, and *reversal induction.* Arousal modulation involved reducing arousal for those who were experiencing unpleasantly high levels of arousal as severe anxiety or increasing arousal for those experiencing unpleasantly low levels of arousal as boredom. Reversal inhibition and reversal induction involved those who were experiencing problems reversing or were *stuck* or *trapped* in a particular combination of states (Lafreniere *et al.,* 2001). Put simply, in the former a person is stuck in a given combination of metamotivational states and chooses to participate in certain activities to obtain satisfaction and pleasant hedonic tone within that particular combination. In the latter, everyday life circumstances may force a person into a fixed metamotivational state combination with accompanying unpleasant hedonic tone. The person learns that by undertaking certain activities he or she can create a desirable escape into an alternative state combination, providing relief and pleasant hedonic tone.

Arousal modulation

As Brown (1997) has argued, and research evidence from Chapter 3 has shown, there are those who use exercise to modulate arousal by increasing unpleasantly low levels of arousal. Seheult (1995) described the case of a secondary exercise dependent competitive body builder who used weight training to create a psychological 'high' or 'buzz':

> He said that over the years he had become 'hooked' on the 'buzz' which he experienced on a regular but somewhat unpredictable basis when engaged in using the weight machines. He found this phenomenon very pleasant and it would appear likely that this had become a major reinforcer for continuing to exercise at a consistently high level. At various times when he decreased the intensity of training, he had found himself no longer able to achieve the 'buzz', thus he had come to the conclusion that there was a minimal level of training which he had to maintain ...
>
> (Seheult, 1995, p. 42)

This quote is a good example of someone who uses intensive exercise to increase arousal. It is interesting that Seheult (1995) pointed to the reinforcing effect of his pleasurable reward for the continuation of his exercise behaviour in the way that Brown (1997) suggested in his model.

Other exercisers use exercise to modulate arousal by decreasing unpleasantly high levels of arousal. A 38-year-old primary exercise dependent individual (Leo) in Blaydon's (2001) qualitative study constitutes a good example of someone who used exercise to reduce arousal and relieve a severe anxiety problem. Over the previous year, Leo had been suffering from anxiety attacks. At the time of the interview, he was running six days and 55 miles per week, but he expected to increase this to 80–90 miles per week. He was a hard worker, with long and irregular hours as a sound balancer in the TV industry, a job that he considered inherently stressful. He had been in the job for nearly 20 years, but in the period before the interview the stress began to affect him for the first time and he started having anxiety problems. He described himself as having a very vulnerable and sensitive personality that he thought he hid by coming across as being confident, cool and conscientious on the outside. He also said that he could be quite a nervous person who tended to keep to himself and liked to keep things constant because he did not like change very much. When asked at interview how his anxiety condition was, he responded:

> I am generally much better with the anxiety and have been discharged from my doctor and I am now free of medication (Paroxtene). I generally tend to consider my condition as a case of 'over-sensitized nerves' rather than panic or anxiety. This follows a period of coming to terms and understanding my condition, its possible causes and its symptoms.

When asked what triggered his anxiety, he stated:

> It is certainly linked with mood changes and an almost sub-conscious awareness of not being in control. Exercise acts as a distraction before getting an anxiety attack. I am not sure of the exact trigger but exercise certainly helps. Exercise is something I love to do so I guess it brings me back in control of what I want to do. I normally feel good during exercise, less so during competition but OK after. I always feel I have achieved a goal, however short that may be, until I need to fulfil it again . . . Exercise really calms me down, relieves my stress which I am guilty of bottling up inside.
>
> (Blaydon, 2001, pp. 115–17)

These quotes demonstrate how exercise was used as an effective strategy for dealing with the unpleasant hedonic tone associated with anxiety attacks. The experience of this particular exerciser provides support for research findings from the exercise psychology literature on the use of exercise for anxiety reduction and for changing unpleasant moods (e.g. Biddle and Mutrie, 2001; Thayer et al., 1994). The use of exercise to modulate arousal in this way is also in accord with Brown's (1997) notion of managing hedonic tone. However, rather than increasing arousal as occurs in some other addictions such as gambling, in this case the modulation is aimed at decreasing unpleasant levels of arousal and anxiety.

In terms of reversal theory, it is clear that the type of work Leo was engaged in was totally mismatched with his telic, arousal avoiding, sympathetic personality and it is perhaps, therefore, not surprising that he experienced stress. The origin of his stress and negative hedonic tone was a feeling of lack of control associated with irregular hours and frequent change that he experienced in his work situation. His inability to achieve a perception of being in control at work resulted in a discrepancy between the level of felt transactional outcome he actually experienced and the level he would like to have experienced. This discrepancy was one source of his tension stress, but it was exacerbated by the experience of high levels of unpleasant felt arousal experienced as anxiety in the telic and conformist states. This gave rise to further increases in negative hedonic tone and tension stress.

By investing in exercise in his efforts to cope with this stress, he had learned that it gave him the possibility of both reducing anxiety and feeling calm post-exercise (related to the telic and conformist states), and the perception of regaining his feelings of control (autic-mastery). This involved reducing unpleasant levels of arousal and improving felt transactional outcome. Exercise also provided a way of improving hedonic tone through the satisfaction of achieving his telic-oriented exercise goals. Thus, there were three different elements to this primary dependent exerciser's coping response to stress.

Leo's plan to increase his running from 55 miles to 80–90 miles per week and to exercise for longer periods (or with greater intensity) might also be an indication that he was becoming tolerant to his current level of exercise activity. It is likely that his hedonic management strategy was becoming less effective and it was becoming necessary for him to do more to achieve the same post-exercise levels of enhanced hedonic tone.

Yates (1991) provided a description of an exerciser whose experience is remarkably similar:

> Max was a dedicated swimmer who also ran. When he moved where there was no swimming pool, he began to escalate his mileage and he continued to increase it over the next three years. He would like to run 60 miles a week. Through running he has become more controlled and he has a greater degree of control over his life. Running compensates for his lack of mastery over his job and relationships. If he is upset, increasing his mileage or pace makes him feel good again. He can push his problems out by running and then he feels cleansed.
>
> (Yates, 1991, p. 34)

The use of exercise to obtain a feeling of control was a theme emphasized in many of the interviews with dependent exercisers (Chapter 7) and emerged as a major dimension in the Bamber *et al.* (2000b, 2003) and Cox and Orford (2004) studies.

Reversal inhibition

Murgatroyd and Apter (1984, 1986) used the term *reversal inhibition* to describe the situation where an individual becomes 'stuck', 'locked' or 'trapped' in a particular metamotivational state or state combination. When this occurs,

reversals become difficult and the individual experiences only very occasional reversals to other states. Miller (1985) was one of the first to recognize
that this reversal problem might be a cause of addictions. It is interesting that
similar terminology (e.g. 'stuck', 'locked', or 'rigid') has been used by both
researchers and some of the participants in their studies to describe the
behaviour of dependent exercisers. For example, Yates (1991) described the
group of 'obligatory' runners that became a focus of her team's research:

> A few of the men stood out from the rest and were identified by other
> runners as different. Instead of the sport contributing to their adaptation,
> running had become their adaptation. They seemed locked into and
> controlled by the activity.
>
> (Yates, 1991, p. 26)

Bamber *et al.* (2000b) provided an example of a secondary exercise
dependent exerciser: 'Meg's exercising was highly regimented. She described
her routine as, "very rigid, and I get very upset if I am thrown out by it"'
(Bamber *et al.*, 2000b, p. 428).

Cox and Orford (2004) wrote about the structure and routine of a primary
exercise dependent exerciser:

> Henry . . . has imposed his own structure to his exercise. He keeps
> diaries as an external sign of the structure and his routines also impose
> structure on his family life. He appears to suggest that this is desirable
> and yet uses a metaphor 'locked' which suggests trapped within the
> routine. This relates to his earlier comment 'I have to do it', suggesting
> the structure is both comforting and confining:
>
> Henry – 'it's like any routine . . . you get locked into it and stop thinking
> about it . . . my whole family know that I get up with the kids on
> Sunday morning give them their breakfast then go for a run . . . that's
> what I do.'
>
> (Cox and Orford, 2004, pp. 177–8)

These quotes indicate that addicted exercisers can become locked into a
particular pattern of behaviour, but does this mean that they are locked in
particular metamotivational states in everyday life and have problems
reversing, as conceptualized in the term reversal inhibition? Although it
should not be assumed that the same behaviour is always accompanied by
the same operative states (Apter, 1982), some tentative conclusions can be
drawn. The overall evidence from the interview studies indicates that, for
dependent exercisers, exercise is the most important feature of their lives.
They are very serious about their exercise, they always try to complete their
goals for the exercise session, and they enjoy the feelings of having personal
control, strength and competence associated with exercising. It might,
therefore, be concluded that dependent exercisers are trapped in a telic-

conformist-autic-mastery state combination and exercise gives them a way to obtain satisfaction in these states. Reversal inhibition has been influential in their becoming addicted to exercise. Linking reversal inhibition to Brown's (1997) seventh proposition about established addictions, it can be seen that management of hedonic tone for these individuals has become extremely limited. It is only when certain states are operative (telic-conformist-autic-mastery) and felt arousal and felt transactional outcome are at appropriate levels that they can alleviate unpleasant negative mood and achieve the positive experience and enhanced hedonic tone that they constantly seek through exercise.

Reversal induction

Some dependent exercisers may be addicted to exercise because inducing reversals through exercise has become their only way of 'unlocking' themselves from particular metamotivational states and counteracting reversal inhibition in daily life. Participants' reports of changes in certain emotions, or, for example, relief from depression after engaging in an exercise regimen, might be indicative of reversals having taken place. Yates (1991) reported the case of a 37-year-old physician with a flourishing practice who ran 70 miles per week and who was driven to achieve his time and distance goals. Dick had been running for ten years and had suffered several major injuries, including one knee injury that required surgery:

> Dick describes himself as a workaholic who has trouble sitting down and relaxing . . . Dick has been married three times. He has been in counselling because of depression, anger, and problems with relationships. These difficulties improved once he began to run. As he increased his running, his need for therapy diminished; he felt mellower and his relationships became more comfortable and more meaningful . . . Dick is a good runner; running harnesses his restlessness and stabilizes his emotional state.
>
> (Yates, 1991, pp. 31–2)

The fact that Dick described himself as a workaholic, with a workaholic's typically intense task-, goal- and performance-oriented approach to life, suggests that he is likely to be stuck in the telic, autic and mastery states. After taking up exercise, Dick's psychological problems diminished; exercise acted as a means of coping with the stress of his workaholic approach to his occupation. Yates' (1991) implicit conclusion is that taking part in exercise promoted specific changes in Dick's psychological make up. Based on reversal theory conceptualizations, it might be speculated that Dick's running activities must have generally reduced his level of arousal (anger is a high arousal emotion associated with the telic-negativistic state combination) and likely sparked reversals among the somatic and transactional states, helping to relieve his negative hedonic tone. It appears that exercise allowed Dick to experience other states more easily. For example, the change in the nature of his relationships with others suggests that the alloic and sympathy states, rather than the autic and mastery states, were more often operative as a result of his exercise activity.

Suggestions for helping exercise dependent individuals

To this point, only the first seven propositions or stages of Brown's (1997) model have been considered. Brown also included three propositions that deal with the process involved in combating established addictions or 'reversing the process' as he termed it. He labelled these propositions 'redistribution and dispersal of the sources of pleasure and reward', 'risk of reversion to the full motivational monopoly' and 'vulnerability to reinstatement of former patterns of reward'.

Once the addict has made a commitment to change his or her addictive behaviour, redistribution and dispersal require sweeping changes in the policy and management of hedonic tone, with a view to reducing or extinguishing the addictive activity (Brown, 1997). The addict needs to become more aware of, and more vigilant about the reinforcement processes involved in his or her behaviour and to make improvements to personal decision-making in other areas of life such as work, recreation, social contacts and daily living. The addict also needs to become more tolerant of short periods of unpleasant hedonic tone, and attempts must be made to discover, revive or rediscover as wide a range of other easily accessible rewarding activities as possible. If this can be achieved, it should allow better personal planning for the manipulation of hedonic tone over the medium and long term, and also help with short-term planning. Producing effective changes in the policy and style of hedonic tone management may take several years (Brown, 1997).

Changing an addicted exerciser's behaviour will not be easy because it has become so crucial to the procurement of good hedonic tone in the person's life, and has been reinforced so strongly as a source of pleasure, that the behaviour will very likely be difficult to extinguish. Cutting down on exercise will be the hardest thing for addicted exercisers to do, as they are strongly motivated to do more rather than less. However, cutting down slightly and taking part in activities other than a person's primary exercise activity, perhaps as part of alternating sports in cross-training, may prove beneficial. Changing the time of day for exercise may also help to break up fixed exercise routines. By including a rest day in exercise schedules, addicted exercisers may come to realize that having some rest allows the body to recover, aches and pains may decrease somewhat and they may even feel better as a result. Taking part with other people in partner or team activities, rather than exercising alone, could help to vary routines and to build or rebuild social relationships that may have been sacrificed in the past due to exercise commitments. Eventually, rest days and free time can be used to discover new, or rediscover old sources of pleasure (e.g. the pleasure of trying new sport activities and/or the pleasure of social interaction) and thus develop ways to manipulate hedonic tone on a broader basis, not restricted only to exercise activity. The idea is to try and break the fixed patterns of the addicted exerciser's motivation and behaviour and make it more varied and interesting by introducing other sources of reward that can provide the same levels of pleasure and intensity of experience that were formerly provided by exercise. Due to the general health benefits accruing from exercise, severely reducing the addict's excessive exercise may be preferable to extinction. However, maintaining involvement in exercise activities may mean that the former addict will be constantly under the threat of reverting to excessive levels of exercise, with the reinstatement of former patterns of reward and exercise once again becoming a motivational monopoly.

In reversal theory terms, the processes of redistribution and dispersal as described by Brown can be seen as attempts to change the exercise addict's rigid operative metamotivation and increase the possibility of inducing reversals. For example, starting to give greater priority to other recreational activities may provoke the addict to reverse from the telic to the paratelic state and slowly change the desire to constantly strive to achieve exercise goals. Also, initiating social contact with others may help the exercise addict to reverse from the self-focused autic to the other-focused alloic state and from the mastery to the sympathy state on occasion. This might allow the strong control focus of the exercise activity to be dissipated over time. By taking gradual steps to improve the ease with which reversals occur and break down reversal inhibition, more balance can be brought to an addict's motivational experience and through time reduce the addictive behaviour.

According to Brown (1997), during redistribution and dispersal there is always the possibility that reversion may take place, with the salience of the exercise activity and the former full motivational monopoly becoming restored. The addict's vulnerability to cross-addictions is high during this stage, but decreases with the improvement in the quality and variety of life, as the number of positive experiences rises and the sources of reward become more varied. Brown's (1997) reinstatement proposition points out that, even if redistribution and dispersal works well, a residual vulnerability endures, and therefore the possibility of the exercise addict reverting to highly intense exercise activity remains for a long time.

Professional counselling from a sport and exercise psychologist or other support from family or friends may help addicted exercisers through recovery, although some determined individuals may be able to manage the changes without support. For those with secondary exercise dependence, where the dependence is bound up with an eating disorder, the condition is more complicated, especially in those who use exercise to control their eating behaviour. Although the same sort of tactics for changing their exercise behaviour will still be appropriate, specialist help will be needed to help these individuals to deal with their eating disorders. Therefore, these individuals should only receive counselling from qualified clinical psychologists or sport and exercise psychologists with clinical training.

Closing comments

This book has attempted to draw together the information on exercise dependence available at this time. Brown's (1997) model, supported by reversal theory, was taken from the mainstream study of addictions and used to provide a meaningful explanatory framework for the material presented in this book. Evidence was examined from a number of general exercise research studies to build a case to show that exercise could act to modulate arousal and other metamotivational variables and manipulate hedonic tone in the way that Brown has argued. Exercise dependence and its connection to eating disorders were explored in detail, in order to provide insights into their relationship in secondary exercise dependence where exercise dependence is secondary to an eating disorder. This exploration was extended to include a broad look at different types of sports and how eating disorders affect athletes in secondary exercise dependence where the eating disorder is secondary to exercise dependence. Endurance sports were specifically addressed and competitive athletes in these sports were found to be particularly at risk for developing a combination of exercise dependence and eating disorders. The results of quantitative questionnaire studies provided details of personality factors that are associated with exercise dependence and some differences (as well as some similarities) were found between primary and secondary exercise dependent individuals among samples of general sport and exercise activity participants and those from the specific sport of triathlon. In addition, findings from qualitative interview studies were reviewed and substantial evidence was presented for classifying both secondary and primary exercise dependence as addictions. The interview studies' findings were shown to be in close agreement with the propositions of Brown's (1997) model of addictions and consistent with reversal theory. Finally, some general suggestions for counselling those individuals with exercise dependence were explored.

The topic of exercise dependence appears to be receiving more attention in recent years, generating a number of important research studies. It is to be hoped that this trend will continue, but, as pointed out in Chapter 7, the present authors have concerns about the Exercise Dependence Questionnaire (EDQ; Ogden *et al.*, 1997) and the way it has been used as a means of identifying those with exercise dependence. Those qualitative studies that used interview techniques appear to have provided richer and more accurate information about exercise dependence and provided some strong guidelines for future research. However, interview-based research also has its limitations. The data obtained often depends on the questions asked in interview and the way those answers are interpreted, which often vary depending on the aims of the researchers. Unless alternative, perhaps innovative forms of research can be utilized, interview-based research may be the best way forward for future research in exercise dependence.

This book is just a beginning. It is some 16 years since the publication of Yates' (1991) book on obligatory exercisers and eating disorders and 12 years since Veale's (1995) publication on primary exercise dependence. While more about exercise dependence is now known, there is still a good deal of further work to be done before it is fully understood.

References

Apter, M. J. (1982) *The experience of motivation*, London: Academic Press.

Apter, M. J. (ed.) (2001) *Motivational styles in everyday life: A guide to reversal theory*, Washington DC: American Psychological Association.

Apter, M. J., Mallows, R. and Williams, S. (1998) 'The development of the Motivational Style Profile', *Personality and Individual Differences*, 24, 7–18.

Bamber, D., Cockerill, I. M. and Carroll, D. (2000a) 'The pathological status of exercise dependence', *British Journal of Sports Medicine*, 34, 125–32.

Bamber, D., Cockerill, I. M., Rodgers, S. and Carroll, D. (2000b) '"It's exercise or nothing": A qualitative analysis of exercise dependence', *British Journal of Sports Medicine*, 34, 423–30.

Bamber, D., Cockerill, I. M., Rodgers, S. and Carroll, D. (2003) 'Diagnostic criteria for exercise dependence in women', *British Journal of Sports Medicine*, 37, 393–400.

Biddle, S. J. H. and Mutrie, N. (2001) *Psychology of physical activity*, London: Routledge.

Blaydon, M. J. (2001) *Descriptive and metamotivational characteristics of primary and secondary exercise dependent and eating disordered participants in intense physical activity*, unpublished doctoral dissertation, Hong Kong: The University of Hong Kong, China.

Blaydon, M. J., Lindner, K. J. and Kerr, J. H. (2002) 'Metamotivational characteristics of eating-disordered and exercise-dependent triathletes', *Psychology of Sport and Exercise*, 3, 223–36.

Blaydon, M. J., Lindner, K. J. and Kerr, J. H. (2004) 'Metamotivational characteristics of exercise dependence and eating disorders in highly active amateur sport participants', *Personality and Individual Differences*, 36, 1419–32.

Brown, R. I. F. (1988) 'Reversal theory and subjective experience in the explanation of addiction and relapse', in M. J. Apter, J. H. Kerr and M. P. Cowles (eds) *Progress in reversal theory*, Amsterdam: Elsevier, 191–212.

Brown, R. I. F. (1997) 'A theoretical model of behavioural addictions – Applied to offending', in J. E. Hodge, M. McMurran and C. R. Hollin (eds) *Addicted to crime?*, New York: Wiley, 13–65.

Brown, R. I. F. (2001) 'Addictions', in M. J. Apter (ed.) *Motivational styles in everyday life: A guide to reversal theory*, Washington DC: American Psychological Association, 155–65.

Cox, R. and Orford, J. (2004) 'A qualitative study of the meaning of exercise for people who could be labelled as "addicted" to exercise – Can "addiction" be applied to high frequency exercising? *Addiction Research and Theory*, 12, 167–88.

Downes, S. (1998) 'Running on empty', *Running Times*, October, 53–6.

Griffiths, M. (1997) 'Exercise addiction: A case study', *Addiction Research and Theory*, 5, 161–8.

Hulley, A. J. and Hill, A. J. (2001) 'Eating disorders and health in elite woman distance runners', *International Journal of Eating Disorders*, 30, 312–17.

Kerr, J. H. and Kuk, G. (2001) 'The effects of low and high intensity exercise on emotions stress and effort', *Psychology of Sport and Exercise*, 2, 173–86.

Kerr, J. H. and van den Wollenberg, A. E. (1997) 'High and low intensity exercise and psychological mood states', *Psychology & Health*, 12, 603–18.

Kerr, J. H. and Vlaswinkel, E.H. (1993) 'Self-reported mood and running', *Work & Stress*, 7, 161–77.

Keski-Rahkonen, A. (2001) 'Exercise dependence – A myth or a real issue?', *European Eating Disorders Review*, 9, 279–83.

Lafreniere, K. D., Ledgerwood, D. M. and Murgatroyd, S. J. (2001) 'Psychopathology, therapy and counseling', in M. J. Apter (ed.) *Motivational styles in everyday life: A guide to reversal theory*, Washington DC: American Psychological Association, 263–85.

Long, C., Smith, J., Midgley, M. and Cassidy, T. (1993) 'Over-exercising in anorexic and normal samples: Behavior and attitudes', *Journal of Mental Health*, 2, 321–7.

Miller, W. R. (1985) 'Addictive behaviour and the theory of psychological reversals', *Addictive Behaviors*, 10, 177–80.

Murgatroyd, S. and Apter, M. J. (1984) 'Eclectic psychotherapy: A structural phenomenological approach', in W. R. Dryden (ed.) *Individual psychotherapy in Britain*, London: Harper & Row, 389–414.

Murgatroyd, S. and Apter, M. J. (1986) 'A structural-phenomenological approach to eclectic psychotherapy', in J. Norcross (ed.) *Casebook of eclectic psychotherapy*, New York: Bruner/Mazel, 260–80.

Ogden, J., Veale, D. M. W. and Summers, Z. (1997) 'The development and validation of the Exercise Dependence Questionnaire', *Addiction Research*, 5, 343–56.

Redican, B. and Hadley, D. S. (1988) 'A field studies project in a city health and leisure club', *Sociology of Sport Journal*, 5, 50–62.

Seheult, C. (1995) 'Hooked on the "buzz": History of a body-building addict', in J. Annett, B. Cripps and H. Steinberg (eds) *Exercise addiction: Motivation for participation in sport and exercise*, Leicester: The British Psychological Society, 41–2.

Sundgot-Borgen, J. (1993) 'Prevalence of eating disorders in female elite athletes', *International Journal of Sport Nutrition*, 3, 29–40.

Sundgot-Borgen, J. (1994a) 'Eating disorders in female athletes', *Sports Medicine*, 17, 176–88.

Sundgot-Borgen, J. (1994b) 'Risk and trigger factors for the development of eating disorders in female elite athletes', *Medicine and Science in Sports and Exercise*, 26, 414–19.

Thayer, R. E., Newman, J. R. and McClain, T. M. (1994) 'The self-regulation of mood: Strategies for changing a bad mood, raising energy, and reducing tension', *Journal of Personality and Social Psychology*, 67, 910–25.

Trimpop, R. M., Kerr, J. H. and Kirkcaldy, B. (1999) 'Comparing personality constructs of risk-taking behavior', *Personality and Individual Differences*, 26, 237–54.

Veale, D. (1995) 'Does primary exercise dependence really exist?', in J. Annett, B. Cripps and H. Steinberg (eds) *Exercise addiction: Motivation for participation in sport and exercise*, Leicester: The British Psychological Society, 1–5.

Yates, A. (1991) *Compulsive exercise and the eating disorders*, New York: Brunner Mazel.

Zuckerman, M. (1979) *Sensation seeking: Beyond the optimal level of arousal*, Hillsdale NJ: Erlbaum.

Appendix A
Getting started with reversal theory[1]

Step 1 in getting started with reversal theory is to note that reversal theory is a *general theory* of psychology that utilizes a *structural phenomenological* approach. In addition, the theory considers human behaviour to be inherently inconsistent and argues that *reversals* between paired *metamotivational states* form the basis of human personality, emotion and motivation (see Figure A.1). Step 2 involves examining the basic features of reversal theory, and the technical terms they have been assigned, in more detail. Where examples have been provided to illustrate concepts from reversal theory, they have been taken from athletes' experience in sport.

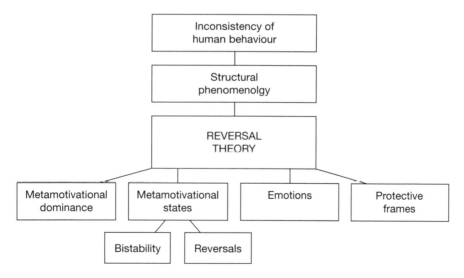

Figure A.1 The main concepts in reversal theory

Source: J. H. Kerr (1994) *Understanding soccer hooliganism* (© 1994 Open University Press). Reproduced with the kind permission of the Open University Press/McGraw-Hill Publishing

Structural phenomenology

Phenomenology is one of the major approaches in the study of psychology. It concentrates on the individual's subjective experience of life events. Structural phenomenology is the special form of phenomenology that is utilized by reversal theory. In structural phenomenology, the subjective experience of cognition and emotion, as well as one's own motivation, is thought to be influenced by certain structures and patterns. Thus, structural phenomenology provides a perspective on how human motivation is organized. Tied in with the individual focus of reversal theory is the notion that there is an inherent inconsistency in the way that people behave. In other words, an athlete who finds him or herself in the same situation on different occasions may behave in totally different ways.

Metamotivational states and reversals

Metamotivational states are mental states that are concerned with how athletes experience their motives. There are eight different metamotivational states bonded together in four pairs that co-exist separately within *bistable systems*. The concept of bistability has been adopted by reversal theory from cybernetics to explain the rapid changes or psychological reversals that take place backwards and forwards over time between any pair of metamotivational states. In cybernetics, a bistable system is one that tends to maintain a specified variable, despite external disturbance, within one or another of two ranges of values of the variable concerned. The four sets of partner metamotivational states are known as the *telic and paratelic, negativistic and conformist, autic and alloic* and *mastery and sympathy* states. The first four are primarily concerned with the way an athlete experiences his or her own bodily arousal and are therefore known as the *somatic states*. The latter four states are primarily concerned with interactions with other people or, in some situations, objects (e.g. motorcycles, boats, horses, skis and other sports equipment), and have therefore been labelled the *transactional states*. In reversal theory, the relative importance of one state over the others at any particular time is known as *salience*. Figure A.2 summarizes the major characteristics of the somatic and transactional metamotivational states.

An analogy might be useful in illustrating the relationship that exists between partner metamotivational states. For example, consider a viewer who is particularly interested in sport sitting down to watch television. Two sports events (e.g. track-and-field athletics and tennis) are being transmitted on different channels – say channels 1 and 2 – at the same time. Although interested in both events, the person concerned can only watch athletics on channel 1 or tennis on channel 2 at any one time, but by using the remote control to switch back and forth between channels, the viewer can see the best action from both events. Here, channel 1 can be thought of as representing one metamotivational state (e.g. the telic state) and channel

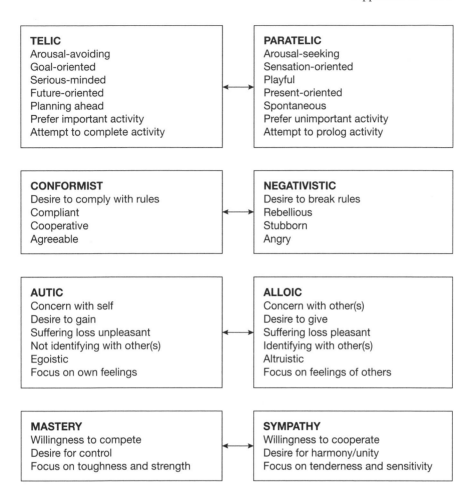

Figure A.2 Characteristics of the four pairs of metamotivational states

2 its paired partner (e.g. the paratelic state), and the switches between channels can be thought of as the reversals that occur between metamotivational states in everyday life (see Figure A.3).

Characteristics of the somatic states

Telic state

With the telic state operative, an athlete's behaviour is likely to be serious, goal oriented and future related in the sense that it involves considerable planning ahead. This form of behaviour is typical of many training situations where a high work rate and the completion of training goals are to the fore. Also, when in this state, athletes will generally have a preference for experiencing low levels of *felt arousal*.

Paratelic state

With the paratelic state operative, an athlete's behaviour is likely to be spontaneous, impulsive and sensation oriented, and geared to prolonging the immediate enjoyment of ongoing activities. In this state, the athlete prefers high levels of felt arousal and, where goals exist, their purpose is to add to the pleasure in a situation. Scandinavian fartlek distance running training is a good example, where fun is the main objective and distance and time are of lesser importance.

Negativistic state

Athletes in the negativistic state tend to be rebellious, stubborn and defiant, feeling the need to act against something or someone. With this state operative, an athlete might react to the aggressive barracking of rival fans and respond by directing a provocative gesture at them.

Conformist state

Athletes in the conformist state are usually agreeable and cooperative and have a desire to comply with rules. The written and unwritten rules and conventions of many sports require compliance by the athletes concerned and, as a result, athletes will often be in the conformist state when competing.

Characteristics of the transactional states

Autic state

The focus for individuals in the autic state is themselves and what happens to them personally in any sporting or other interaction. If an athlete perceives him or herself as successful in an interaction, it is a pleasant experience; if unsuccessful, it is experienced as unpleasant. A try-saving tackle in rugby or a diving catch in the cricket outfield executed successfully would engender pleasant feelings for an athlete with the autic state operative.

Alloic state

When the alloic state is operative, the focus for an athlete is what happens to other athletes, coaching staff, or even officials in any sporting interaction. Perceiving these other participants as having been successful will induce feelings of pleasure and satisfaction in that particular athlete. For example, for a player in the alloic state, a winning goal scored by a field hockey teammate in injury time at the end of a close, hard-fought game would be experienced in this way.

Mastery state

Athletes may often find themselves in the mastery state when competing against another athlete or team. In the usual competitive situation, they will feel the need to be tough and masterful in order to defeat opponents.

Sympathy state

When the sympathy state is operative, athletes will feel the need to empathize with others, perhaps teammates or supporting spectators. Here feelings of harmony and unity may be important.

How reversals take place

Reversals are thought to be involuntary and sometimes unexpected. In other words, a person cannot suddenly decide that he or she would prefer to be in, say, the telic state and consciously prompt a reversal to that state from the paratelic state. Reversal theory hypothesizes that there are three ways in which reversals take place. These have been termed *contingency*, *frustration* and *satiation* (see Figure A.3).

Contingency

A club cricketer plays recreational cricket at the weekend. He is the team's best fast bowler and takes his bowling very seriously, thinking about and

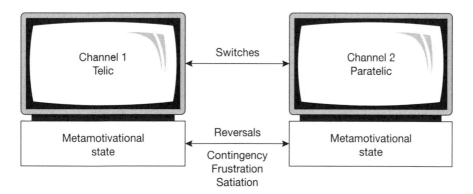

Figure A.3 Television channel switching illustrating how reversals are induced by the three types of inducing agents

planning the series of balls in each over very carefully. When he is bowling, he is typically in the telic state. However, he has never shown much talent or skill with the bat and he regularly bats near the bottom of the team batting order. As a result, his attitude when batting has been to treat it as a bit of a laugh, getting to the crease and swinging his bat with reckless abandon, hoping to notch up a few lucky runs before he gets bowled out. When he is batting he is typically in the paratelic state.

During one particular match in the latter stages of a cup competition, his more talented teammates at the top and middle of the batting order fail to come to terms with a very skilful spin bowler and they are skittled out for a very low score. He finds himself going out to bat with nine wickets down. He and his partner are the last batsmen. Usually when he bats he is in the paratelic state, but now, owing to the sudden collapse of his team's normally dependable batting and the fact that he has to bat slowly and cautiously to try and achieve a good score and get his team out of trouble, he undergoes a reversal and finds himself in the telic state. In this example, the batting collapse is an environmental event that has induced a reversal from the paratelic to the telic state (e.g. Svebak *et al.*, 1982).

Frustration

A rugby league match involves two teams from a premier division, but with players of very different abilities and playing styles. One team has extremely skilful players who are intent on playing the game to the best of their ability and using team strategy and tactics that involve a flowing, entertaining game. The other team's players are not as skilful and have developed a style of play that is dependent on 'mixing it' with the opposing players and trying to upset their playing style. This often means using physically violent, unlawful tactics that they have employed with some success in previous matches.

Towards the end of the first half of the game, a forward from the skilful team receives the ball and runs at speed, trying to break through the opposition defence. He is tackled by two defenders. One of the defenders has tackled low and taken the attacking forward around the legs. The second defender has tackled around the upper body and, just as the players hit the ground, he elbows the attacker hard in the face. The foul play was unseen by referee and touch judges. In addition, the opposition has been using very dubious tactics since the start of the game, preventing the attacking team from playing their usual open style of play. This is the third or fourth time that the attacking forward has been subjected to foul play. Following the instructions of the team coach, he has not reacted to the previous incidents, remaining in the conformist state and adhering to the coach's instructions and the rules of the game. With the latest incident, however, a reversal from the conformist to the negativistic state takes place, prompted by the repeated acts of foul play. The attacking forward angrily retaliates and a punch-up between the two players develops. This time, however, the touch judge has observed the retaliation and, after consulting with the referee, the attacking forward (feeling even more aggrieved and negativistic) is sent off the pitch to the 'sin bin'. This example illustrates the second type of reversal induction, where a reversal has occurred due to conditions of *frustration*, where an athlete has been unable to obtain satisfaction in an operative state or state combination (see, for example, Barr *et al.*, 1990).

Satiation

A professional volleyball player is a member of a team based in Japan. Prior to the start of the playing season, she participates in pre-season training and attends a special summer training camp. Once the season begins, she becomes a permanent member of the team and plays in all the team's matches. She has a very serious and dedicated approach to volleyball and when she is training and playing she usually has the telic state operative. At the end of a long season, she joins her national team at a four-day international tournament. During her last game, at a stage when the two opposing teams are evenly matched, she suddenly reverses from the telic to the paratelic state. She finds herself in a rather playful mood, making unplanned, spontaneous plays. Even so, her team manages to win and returns to the dressing room. After showering and changing, the player, still with the paratelic state operative, leaves the volleyball facility and goes out on the town for an all-night binge of drinking and partying with some of her teammates. This example illustrates the third type of reversal-inducing agent, *satiation*, which is increasingly likely to induce a reversal if an athlete has been in one metamotivational state for some time (e.g. Lafreniere *et al.*, 1988).

Although reversals are thought to be involuntary, some research evidence does suggest that people may be able to place themselves in particular situations and contexts, or create environmental conditions that are likely to induce reversals to particular metamotivational states (e.g. Kerr and Tacon, 1999). Some examples of research that examined reversals in sport are: Cox and Kerr (1989, 1990), research on competitive squash; Kerr and Vlaswinkel (1993), a study on long distance running; and Males and Kerr (1996), research on slalom canoeing. Details of these studies and other reversal theory sport research can be found in Kerr (1997, 1999).

Metamotivational dominance

To return to the television analogy used earlier, if the action is especially thrilling, a viewer may spend more time watching one channel than the other. In a similar way, though psychological reversals between metamotivational states are thought to take place frequently, each athlete will vary in the amount of time spent in either one of two partner states. Athletes who have a tendency or innate bias to spend more time in one metamotivational state over its partner are said to be, for example, *telic dominant* or *mastery dominant*. Even though athletes may exhibit particular state dominances, they will reverse and spend time in their non-dominant states.

Research examining metamotivational dominance in sport has shown, for example, that telic dominance is associated with participation in and preference for endurance sports, such as long distance running and hiking (Svebak and Kerr, 1989), and paratelic dominance with explosive sports such as baseball and cricket (Svebak and Kerr, 1989), as well as risk sports such as parachuting, motorcycle racing and snowboarding (Cogan and Brown, 1998; Kerr, 1991).

Protective frames and parapathic emotions

A *protective frame* is a kind of psychological bubble or, more specifically, a phenomenological frame that provides a sense of safety in dangerous situations or circumstances. This produces a paradox of danger-that-is-not-danger and allows people to enjoy pleasant high arousal associated with arousal seeking in the paratelic state (Apter, 1993, p. 31). There are three main types of protective frames, known as the *confidence, safety-zone* and *detachment* frames: The confidence frame provides feelings of safety in the face of risk through confidence in one's skills and those of others and the dependability of equipment; the safety-zone frame provides feelings of safety through the perception that in fact there is no source of threat; and the detachment frame provides feelings of safety through the fact that one is merely an observer (Apter, 2001, p. 47). Confidence and safety-zone frames are most important for athletes when performing, and safety-zone and detachment frames are most important for spectators and fans when watching sporting contests.

In special circumstances, where a paratelic protective frame exists, high arousal emotions that are usually experienced as unpleasant in the telic state (e.g. anxiety, anger) can be experienced as pleasant. In this form they are known as *parapathic emotions*. Parapathic emotions can be experienced in any of the safety-zone, confidence or detachment frames, and they then take on a special nature. Apter, describing the special quality of parapathic emotions stated:

> Nevertheless the reversal theory thesis is that *all* high arousal emotions, however unpleasant in the telic state, can be experienced in some form in the paratelic state, and that they will always be pleasant in this state. However, to be experienced in the paratelic state without a reversal to the telic state occurring, these normally telic emotions have to undergo a type of transformation, the result of which is that they come to have in the paratelic state a special phenomenological quality which differentiates them quite clearly from the corresponding emotions in the telic state.
>
> (Apter, 1982, p. 109)

According to reversal theory, it is by means of paratelic protective frames that recreational or competitive athletes involved in risk sports, such as skydiving, are able to enjoy activities that others perceive as highly dangerous. The skydiver, for example, can experience the unpleasant telic anxiety typically associated with skydiving in a pleasant form, through paratelic protective frames and parapathic emotions. Of course, if for any reason the frame should break (for example, as a result of a sudden equipment failure), the pleasant parapathic emotion (anxiety) will once again be experienced in its unpleasant form. Experiencing protective frames is synonymous with being in the paratelic state. Kerr (1997) has explored the reversal theory concept of protective frames and participation in dangerous sports, and Apter (1992/2006) has explored the concept across the whole gamut of sport, recreational and other activities.

Metamotivational state combinations

Step 3 in getting started with reversal theory is to examine a more complex development, that of *metamotivational state combinations* and the emotions that occur as a result.

Two-way somatic state combinations

Perhaps the best way of illustrating the concept of metamotivational state combinations is to return to the television analogy. The original setup can be extended to include two more channels. There are now four channels available to the viewer: channels 1, 2, 3 and 4. With the split-screen function that is available on some contemporary televisions, a viewer can watch two channels at the same time. However, suppose the split-screen function works in such a way that either channel 1 or 2 can be viewed on one panel and either 3 or 4 can be viewed on the other. This would mean that there are four possible split-screen combinations between which a viewer could channel-switch: channels 1 and 3, channels 1 and 4, channels 2 and 3, channels 2 and 4. Here, as well as channel 1 representing the telic state and channel 2 representing the paratelic state, channels 3 and 4 can be thought of as representing the negativistic and conformist metamotivational states, respectively (see Figure A.4). Like the switches between channels, reversals between telic and paratelic states and between negativistic and conformist states are possible, and the different split-screen combinations represent possible metamotivational combinations of the four somatic states (telic-negativistic, telic-conformist, paratelic-negativistic, paratelic-conformist).

Some examples from sport may help to illustrate how these two-way somatic state combinations work. The paratelic-conformist state combination is likely to be operative when a person is playing a leisurely game of pool or snooker with a friend. The game finishes and they decide to play another one. However, the friend suggests that in the next game they should have a

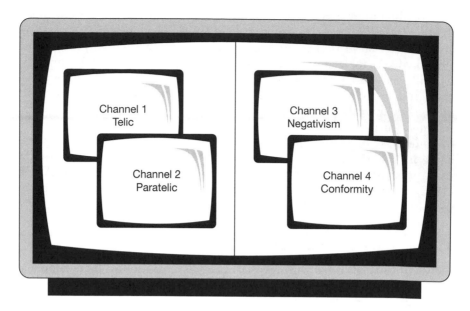

Figure A.4 The television split screen analogy representing two-way somatic state combinations

sizeable wager on the outcome. This changes the players' perception of the seriousness of the play and might well induce a reversal from the paratelic to the telic state. Thus, if a reversal does occur, the person's state combination changes from paratelic-conformity to telic-conformity (conformity because the player has to adhere to the rules and conventions of the game). For professional pool or snooker players involved in top-level competitions, the telic-conformist state combination would be likely to be operative because of the seriousness of the competition and the large amounts of prize money to be won by successful play.

Angry athletes who verbally abuse, push or, very occasionally, strike umpires or referees are likely to be in the telic-negativistic state combination. This usually occurs when the umpire or referee has made what the athlete considers to be an unfair decision against the athlete or the team. The abusive behaviour is a response to perceived injustice.

When athletes' behaviour involves doing something 'just for the hell of it', then it is probable that they are in a paratelic-negativistic state combination. A good example of paratelic-negativism is the ethos of the style of play of the Barbarians rugby team – a specially selected team mostly comprised of players from England, Ireland, Scotland and Wales that plays a one-off match against visiting touring teams from other countries. The Barbarians' tradition is that they play in an unconventional, entertaining way, throwing caution aside and trying personal skills and team moves and tactics that they would rarely try in their regular telic-conformist-oriented matches. In this way, players can, to some extent at least, enjoy defying the usual expectations and break with the established way of doing things.

Two-way transactional state combinations

What is true for the somatic states is also true for the transactional states. Imagine a second set of four channels, again arranged in two pairs (5–6 and 7–8). Channels 5 and 6 represent the autic and alloic states and channels 7 and 8 the mastery and sympathy states, respectively. In the same way as for the four previous channels, four more channel combinations are possible; channels 5 and 7, channels 5 and 8, channels 6 and 7 and channels 6 and 8. (Remember, only 5 or 6 and 7 or 8 can be viewed at any one time.) These channel combinations represent combinations of partner transactional states that produce the autic-mastery, autic-sympathy, alloic-mastery, and alloic-sympathy metamotivational state combinations (see Figure A.5).

To take some more sport examples, many athletes involved in elite-level individual sports (e.g. track-and-field athletic events) will have the autic-mastery state combination operative when they perform. They have dedicated themselves to maximizing their strength and fitness and have mastered their

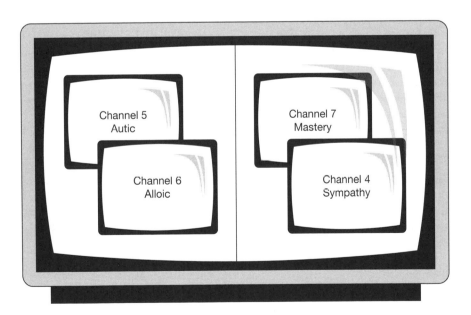

Figure A.5 The television split screen analogy representing two-way transactional state combinations

technique, with a view to defeating their opponents. Their focus is on themselves and being successful, preferably winning. However, a reversal from mastery to sympathy state might occur if the athlete had been unluckily disqualified (e.g. for false-starting, no-throwing or no-jumping). This would result in an autic-sympathy state combination. That is, the athlete would want to be sympathized with and reassured.

Conversely, a male coach guiding his athlete or team through a tournament is likely to be in the alloic-mastery state as he instructs, guides and urges his athlete or team towards victory. The alloic-sympathy state combination might be operative in an athlete who, after competing well, stops at the edge of the playing arena to sign autographs for admiring teenage fans.

Four-way metamotivational combinations

Imagine that the two sets of four channels in the television analogy have been added together and it is now possible for the viewer to watch four channels (one from each pair) at any one time through a four-way split-screen. As shown in Figure A.6, there are four television channels possible in any combination. This means that, for example, channels 1, 3, 5 and 8 could be viewed together, as could channels 2, 3, 6 and 8. These television channel combinations represent the metamotivational state combinations of telic-negativistic-autic-mastery, and paratelic-negativistic-alloic-sympathy, respectively. Of course, these are examples; several other four-way meta-motivational combinations are possible.

Reversals between partner states will occur, and so the component states within any state combination will change relatively frequently. An analogy is real-life cable television, which has one channel consisting of an overview of all the other channels, often showing twelve or more channels in miniature on one regular-sized screen. As the viewer watches, the mini-channels change periodically in an apparently random organization to show brief glimpses of the many cable channels on offer.

This arrangement of metamotivational state combinations is possible through the introduction of the concept of *multistable systems*, which, like the bistable system, also originates from cybernetics. In reversal theory, a multistable system is really a more complex version of the bistable arrangement that exists between any two partner states. The two sets of somatic states and the two sets of transactional states interact within a multistable system. Thus, reversal theory is a multistable theory of motivation.

Four-way state combinations in sport

The Eco Challenge is a long-distance endurance team race over extremely difficult terrain that involves activities such as hiking, running, swimming, mountain biking, canoeing, rock climbing, abseiling and horse riding. The Eco Challenge is designed to be exactly that: a challenge that pushes the

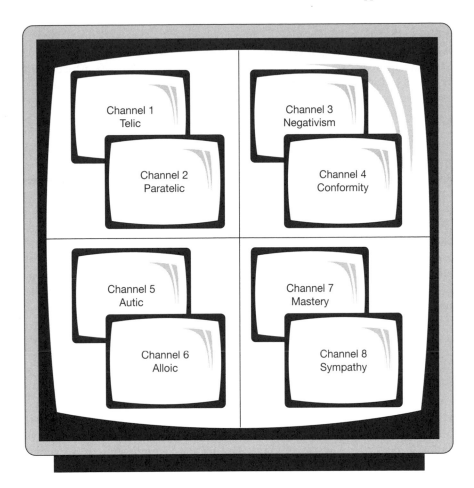

Figure A.6 The television split screen analogy representing four-way somatic and transactional state combinations

competing teams of three men and one woman to their absolute maximum and beyond. Team members voluntarily suffer excruciating pain from blisters, pulled muscles, cramp, injuries from falls, intense heat and cold, dehydration, lack of sleep and other more serious medical conditions. Teams have to plan their own routes over each stage and all the teams in the race are carefully checked at regular rest and food stops. When a team or individual athlete's long-term health or, in some instances, life is threatened, organizers and medical support staff can prevent them from continuing. Back-up helicopters often have to search for competitors in trouble and airlift them back to base hospitals. All four team members have to finish the race; if one is forced to drop out, then the others have to stop as well.

The Eco Challenge provides a useful example of how metamotivational state combinations and reversals might work in the sport context. In an event like this, lasting several days, where athletes repeatedly encounter new and difficult, challenging situations, it is likely that an athlete will experience numerous different metamotivational states and state combinations. For example, when a team is planning their route for the first stage of the race, team members are likely to be in the telic and conformist states. They are also likely to have the alloic and mastery states operative as team cohesion and the desire for their colleagues to be successful is strong. At a later stage, when faced with a long and tricky abseil down a wet and slippery rock face, the athletes may find themselves firmly in a telic-conformist-autic-mastery state combination as they concentrate hard and use all their skill to personally master the task at hand.

At another stage in the race, a tired team member suffering from severe foot problems may reverse from the operative telic and mastery states to the paratelic and sympathy states, as he jokes with medical staff while they treat his cuts and blisters at a rest stop. His overall operative state combination in this situation is likely to be paratelic-conformist-autic-sympathy, with the autic-sympathy combination being most prominent. Once treatment is complete, and as the time to restart the race approaches, the athlete might reverse from paratelic to telic and from sympathy to mastery states in anticipation of what lies ahead.

In a competitive race such as this, the experience of some states may be less common than others. There would, for example, seem to be few occasions for these athletes to have the negativistic state operative. It must also be kept in mind that in a race of this kind, although certain metamotivational combinations may be operative for fairly long periods, reversals are always likely to occur as a result of sudden unexpected environmental events, frustration or satiation. For example, a fall off a mountain bike resulting in severe scrapes and bruises, a slip from a rope while crossing a river resulting in a complete soaking in freezing-cold water, or a canoe capsize in a choppy sea are all unexpected environmental events that might induce reversals. Also, at any one time in a metamotivational state combination, one or two states may predominate over the others. In most of the Eco Challenge race situations, the mastery state may well be salient for many of the competitors.

Metamotivational variables and the sixteen primary emotions

The preference for different levels of felt arousal in the telic and paratelic states has already been mentioned in the subsection 'Characteristics of the somatic states'. Felt arousal is one of reversal theory's *metamotivational variables*, which are associated with the different sets of partner metamotivational states. Felt arousal is the degree to which an athlete feels him or herself to be worked up. Other metamotivational variables include *felt transactional outcome* (transactional states; the degree to which a person feels him or herself to have gained or lost in an interaction); *felt significance* (telic and paratelic states; how much a person perceives a goal he or she is pursuing as significant and serving purposes beyond itself); *felt negativism* (negativistic and conformist states; how much a person feels him or herself to be acting against an external rule or requirement); *felt toughness* (mastery and sympathy states; how much a person feels him or herself to be tough, strong or in control); and *felt identification* (autic and alloic states; how much a person feels him or herself to be egoistic or altruistic).

How different levels of these metamotivational variables are experienced has important implications for an athlete's experience of emotions. In this regard, felt arousal and felt transactional outcome are the two most important metamotivational variables. Felt arousal is a metamotivational variable concerned with the somatic states and its importance in sport has been repeatedly demonstrated by reversal theory sport research (e.g. Cox and Kerr, 1989, 1990; Kerr and Cox, 1989, 1990; Kerr and Vlaswinkel, 1993; Males and Kerr, 1996).

The experience of felt arousal is dependent on whether the conformist or negativistic state is allied with the telic or paratelic state in a two-way combination. An athlete with the telic-conformist state combination operative generally prefers low levels of felt arousal. With the paratelic-conformist state combination operative, high levels of felt arousal are generally preferred. As shown in Figure A.7, the experience of preferred levels of felt arousal is, in both cases, associated with positive hedonic tone and is experienced as pleasant *relaxation* and *excitement*, respectively. Non-preferred high levels of felt arousal in the telic state and low levels of felt arousal in the paratelic state result in negative hedonic tone and are experienced as unpleasant *anxiety* and *boredom*, respectively. Thus there are four possible somatic emotions that may result from the experience of felt arousal conditions in the telic- or paratelic-conformist state combination.

Four additional somatic emotions are experienced when athletes are in the telic- and paratelic-negativistic state combinations. Referring again to Figure A.7, *placidity* and *provocativeness* are the two pleasant emotions and *sullenness* and *anger* the two unpleasant emotions resulting from the various state combinations. In each case, they are also related to the experience of preferred and non-preferred levels of felt arousal, and a reversal between partner states would change the experience of arousal. For example, an athlete might be experiencing unpleasant boredom (paratelic low arousal), but a reversal to the telic state (within a two-way combination with the conformist state) would result in the low arousal then being experienced as pleasant relaxation. Equally, for the two high arousal emotions, unpleasant telic anxiety would be experienced pleasantly as paratelic excitement if a telic to paratelic reversal took place.

Felt transactional outcome is a metamotivational variable concerned with the transactional states. As shown in Figure A.8, a similar series of state combinations between the autic-alloic and mastery-sympathy pairs of states

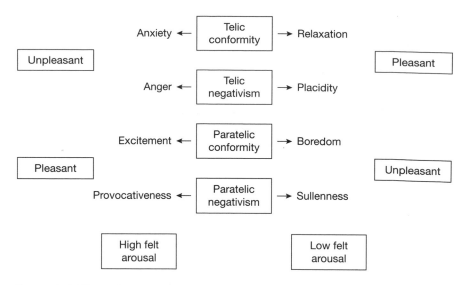

Figure A.7 The eight somatic emotions generated by possible combinations of the telic-paratelic and negativism-conformity pairs of states

Source: J. H. Kerr (1994) *Understanding soccer hooliganism* (© 1994 Open University Press). Reproduced with the kind permission of the Open University Press/McGraw-Hill Publishing

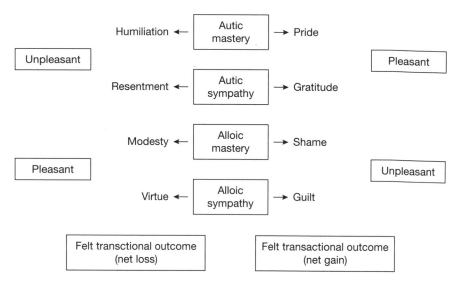

Figure A.8 The eight transactional emotions generated by possible combinations of the autic-alloic and mastery-sympathy pairs of states

Source: J. H. Kerr (1994) *Understanding soccer hooliganism* (© 1994 Open University Press). Reproduced with the kind permission of the Open University Press/McGraw-Hill Publishing

and the experience of felt transactional outcome in terms of net gain or loss result in the experience of eight transactional emotions. These are *pride, modesty, humiliation, shame, gratitude, virtue, guilt and resentment.*

The experience of metamotivational variables in both somatic and transactional state combinations contributes to hedonic tone or experienced pleasure. Provided reversals are not ongoing, athletes at any one time will experience one somatic and one transactional emotion, but the strength of two emotions may vary (for example, a judo player who progresses to the quarterfinals of a tournament after injuring his or her opponent in a throw might experience mild excitement and strong guilt). Overall hedonic tone is, therefore, a composite of the two and reflects the strengths of the contributing emotions. Stress may result from mismatches in preferred and felt levels of the metamotivational variables and is reflected in low levels of hedonic tone and the experience of unpleasant emotions (see Figures A.7 and A.8). The reversal theory approach to stress is explained in the following, final section of the chapter.

Experiencing stress in sport

Step 4 in getting started with reversal theory focuses on how athletes experience stress and how they can attempt to cope with it. As mentioned in the previous section, any mismatch or discrepancy between felt and preferred levels of metamotivational variables, such as felt arousal and felt transactional outcome, will lead to stress. For example, an archer at a competition may typically perform in a specific metamotivational state combination at a preferred level of arousal. If, however, at one particular archery meet, a marked arousal discrepancy occurs between the archer's actual and preferred levels of arousal, the archer is likely to experience stress. In reversal theory, there are two forms or types of stress (Svebak and Apter, 1997). The stress experienced by the archer, caused by a mismatch in preferred and felt arousal levels, is known as *tension stress* and the effort expended by the archer in trying to reduce tension stress is known as *effort stress*. Effort stress is an attempt at coping with discrepancies in levels of metamotivational variables. For example, tension stress and effort stress can be experienced in both telic and paratelic states. In the telic state, tension stress is experienced as unpleasant threat or anxiety, and in the paratelic state it is experienced as unpleasant lack of threat, or boredom. Effort stress in the telic state takes the form of effortful coping, but in the paratelic state it takes the form of responding to challenge(s).

In the case of the archer, let us suppose that the telic state is operative within his or her usual competitive state combination, with accompanying low levels of felt and preferred arousal. The archer will experience telic tension stress if, for example, felt arousal increases as a result of adverse weather conditions during the competition. Increased felt arousal interferes with the archer's pursuance of his or her desired goals and results in unpleasant feelings of anxiety. These unpleasant feelings may lead to effort stress as the archer initiates compensatory coping behaviour aimed at reducing tension and minimizing interference in the archer's attempts at goal achievement.

Conversely, consider the triple jumper whose preferred performance state combination includes the paratelic state with accompanying high felt and preferred arousal. If, for example, at a certain athletics meet, injury forces the withdrawal of the jumper's main rival, the triple jumper's levels of felt arousal may become lower, and the resultant mismatch in arousal levels will be experienced as unpleasant paratelic tension stress. Instead of the competition being challenging and exciting, it is now experienced by the triple jumper as boring. In order to offset the paratelic tension stress, the triple jumper needs to initiate some form of present-oriented coping activity (experienced as paratelic effort stress) in an attempt to increase his or her level of felt arousal. This might take the form of setting up other challenges, such as trying to beat his or her personal best distance, or perhaps making an attempt at a new record.

For an athlete experiencing telic or paratelic tension stress, there are a number of options for manipulating or managing arousal levels, for example through cognitive intervention. Many sport psychology texts (e.g. Morris and Summers, 1995; Murphy, 1995) suggest that an athlete such as the archer above, experiencing anxiety (telic tension stress), could adopt an arousal reduction strategy such as a self-relaxation technique (Jacobson, 1974) to reduce his or her level of felt arousal. However, this type of intervention would be completely counter-productive for an athlete such as the triple jumper, experiencing paratelic tension stress. It is not a lowering of felt arousal that is required in this case, but the opposite, some form of arousal-enhancing strategy aimed at increasing felt arousal levels.

Another effective option for the athlete experiencing telic or paratelic tension stress is not to attempt to modulate felt arousal levels, but to induce a reversal to the partner metamotivational state. This would allow a reinterpretation of arousal levels and a subsequent reduction in tension stress, as any mismatch in felt and preferred arousal levels is corrected. Figure A.9 summarizes the two options for cognitive intervention available to the athlete experiencing either telic or paratelic tension stress.

In the examples used above, felt arousal was the metamotivational variable and telic and paratelic forms of tension stress were discussed. Equally, the other metamotivational variables and other forms of tension stress could have been used. It should be possible to modulate levels of felt transactional outcome and even felt negativism and felt toughness, or induce reversals between the partner states. Prior to the implementation of any of the possible intervention strategies described above, it is essential that the coach and the athlete are able to determine when the performer is experiencing different forms of tension stress.

Incidentally, reversal theory predicts that athletes' stress response may be influenced by their metamotivational dominance. Research by Summers

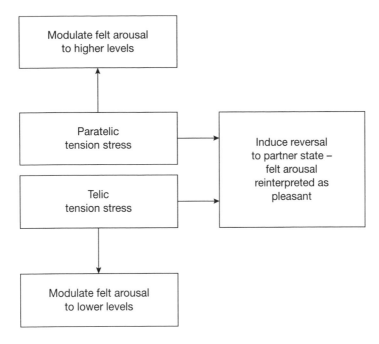

Figure A.9 The four available options for alleviating tension stress

and Stewart (1993), following on from the work of Martin *et al.* (1987), which examined dominance and the stress response in a general non-sport sample, has confirmed this prediction, showing that, while telic dominant athletes prefer low levels of stress, paratelic dominant athletes actually enjoy moderate levels of stress.

Closing comments

If the challenge of summarizing reversal theory in a single chapter has been successful, the reader should now have a good grasp of its basic concepts. For those who already had some knowledge of the theory, it is hoped that this appendix has acted as a kind of refresher course. Appendix A is also a source to be consulted when the need arises as progress is made through the rest of the book.

Note

1   Apart from some minor changes, the contents of Appendix A appeared as Chapter 1 in Kerr, J. H. (2001) *Counselling athletes: Applying reversal theory*, London: Routledge.

References

Apter, M. J. (1982) *The experience of motivation: The theory of psychological reversals*, London: Academic Press.

Apter, M. J. (1992) *The dangerous edge*, New York: Free Press.

Apter, M. J. (1993) 'Phenomenological frames and the paradoxes of experience', in J. H. Kerr, S. Murgatroyd and M. J. Apter (eds) *Advances in reversal theory*, Amsterdam: Swets and Zeitlinger, 27–39.

Apter, M. J. (ed.) (2001) *Motivational styles in everyday life: A guide to reversal theory*, Washington DC: American Psychological Association.

Apter, M. J. (2006) *Danger: Our quest for excitement*, Oxford: Oneworld Publications.

Barr, S. A., McDermott, M. R. and Evans, P. (1990) 'Predicting persistence: A study of telic and paratelic frustration', in J. H. Kerr, S. Murgatroyd and M. J. Apter (eds) *Advances in reversal theory*, Amsterdam: Swets and Zeitlinger, 123–36.

Cogan, N. A. and Brown, R. I. F. (1998) 'Metamotivational dominance, states and injuries in risk and safe sport', *Personality and Individual Differences*, 27, 503–18.

Cox, T. and Kerr, J. H. (1989) 'Arousal effects during tournament play in squash', *Perceptual and Motor Skills*, 69, 1275–80.

Cox, T. and Kerr, J. H. (1990) 'Self-reported mood in competitive squash', *Personality and Individual Differences*, 11, 2, 199–203.

Jacobson, P. (1974) *Progressive relaxation*, Chicago IL: University of Chicago Press.

Kerr, J. H. (1991) 'Arousal-seeking in risk sport participants', *Personality and Individual Differences*, 12, 6, 613–16.

Kerr, J. H. (1994) *Understanding soccer hooliganism*, Buckingham: Open University Press/McGraw-Hill.

Kerr, J. H. (1997) *Motivation and emotion in sport: Reversal theory*, Hove: Psychology Press.

Kerr, J. H. (ed.) (1999) *Experiencing sport: Reversal theory*, Chichester: J. Wiley and Sons.

Kerr, J. H. and Cox, T. (1989) 'Effects of metamotivational dominance and metamotivational state on squash task performance', *Perceptual and Motor Skills*, 67, 171–4.

Kerr, J. H. and Cox, T. (1990) 'Cognition and mood in relation to the performance of a squash task', *Acta Psychologica*, 73, 1, 103–14.

Kerr, J. H. and Tacon, P. (1999) 'Psychological responses to different types of locations and activities', *Journal of Environmental Psychology*, 19, 287–94.

Kerr, J. H. and Vlaswinkel, E. H. (1993) 'Self-reported mood and running', *Work & Stress*, 7, 3, 161–77.

Lafreniere, K., Cowles, M. P. and Apter, M. J. (1988) 'The reversal phenomenon: Reflections on a laboratory study', in M. J. Apter, J. H. Kerr and M. P. Cowles (eds) *Progress in reversal theory*, Amsterdam: North-Holland/Elsevier, 257–66.

Males, J. R. and Kerr, J. H. (1996) 'Stress, emotion and performance in elite slalom canoeists', *The Sport Psychologist*, 10, 17–36.

Martin, R. A., Kuiper, N. A., Olinger, L. J. and Dobbin, J. (1987) 'Is stress always bad? Telic versus paratelic dominance as a stress moderating variable', *Journal of Personality and Social Psychology*, 53, 970–82.

Morris, T. and Summers, J. (1995) *Sport psychology: Theory, applications and issues*, Chichester: J. Wiley and Sons.

Murphy, S. M. (1995) *Sport psychology interventions*, Champaign IL: Human Kinetics.

Summers, J. and Stewart, E. (1993) 'The arousal performance relationship: Examining different conceptions', in S. Serpa, J. Alves, V. Ferriera and A. Paula-Brito (eds) *Proceedings of the VIII World Congress of Sport Psychology*, Lisbon: International Society of Sport Psychology, 229–32.

Svebak, S. and Apter, M. J. (1997) *Stress and health: A reversal theory perspective*, Washington DC: Taylor & Francis.

Svebak, S. and Kerr, J. H. (1989) 'The role of impulsivity in preference for sports', *Personality and Individual Differences*, 10, 1, 51–8.

Svebak, S., Storfjell, O. and Dalen, K. (1982) 'The effect of a threatening context upon motivation and task-induced physiological changes', *British Journal of Psychology*, 73, 505–12.

Author index

Subject index